An
OLD FART'S GUIDE
TO ALMOST
EVERYTHING...
That Matters

WILLIAM B. WADDELL, MD

ISBN: 1469990628
ISBN-13: 9781469990620

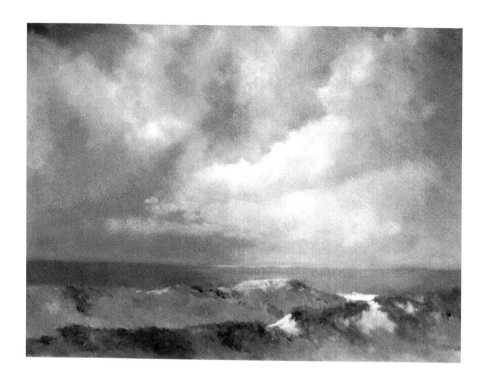

To my fellow Old Farts and to those
whose interest includes becoming one!
And especially these members in my island community;
Thad Wester, Bob Timmons, Bryant Frech, and Brooke
Williams. Thanks to my wife, Emily, and to
Anne Boozell and Bob Helgeson for reviewing
the manuscript and their suggestions.

One more big thank you to Peter Quinn whose thoughtful
illustrations helped bring the book to life.

Contents

Introduction

What's an old fart? Well if you don't know by now you probably can't read this book. You can, of course, look it up on the Internet, or just say, "It takes one to know one".

I do know that older individuals break wind more frequently than anyone else. Maybe we're just not as discreet about it. It's likely, though, that our gut loses some of its ability to break down carbohydrates, allowing them to ferment and make more carbon dioxide, hydrogen, and methane. Like everything else we own, the rectal sphincter gets flabby with age, and we don't control it as well as we used to. Yes, be careful!

Then again, socially speaking, the elder persons, particularly males, probably don't care as much. By the way, this little book pertains primarily to us

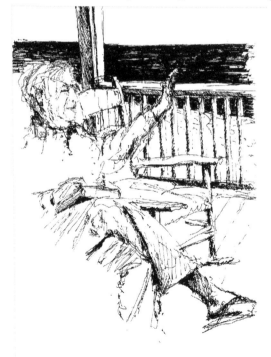

males. Being still of competent mind, I won't presume to speak for women. I have observed, though, that females tend to be more delicate about farting in public places. Be that as it may, we all fart about the same number of times every day. So there.

I know that we all go through this, but it never fails to amaze me when I think about the speed with which time passes as we get older. The slope gets steeper as we get older. Ah well... Days seem like hours, weeks seem like days, months seem like weeks. Who needs a calendar? I can tell that time is passing faster by the speed with which I empty my prescription bottles.

No one likes to be betrayed, especially by our own. But, that's exactly what our body does to us with advancing years. It's one of the unhappy revelations that we all face to one degree or another. In one sense that is what this book is all about.

This book will cover my feelings and opinions about many, if not most, of the things that plague us as we proceed through these golden years. They're golden, of course, because it is so damn expensive to keep us in good health. As a family physician, I thought I knew about all this stuff. Having been fortunate enough to enter my eighth decade, I really know and appreciate these pearls that I am about to cast before you from the most personal aspect. You will not find tables, esoteric statistics, and quotes from scientific studies in this book. There are many places to delve into details, if they are of interest. The Internet has given us an extraordinary ability to do our own research. I have elected to do a general description of the body's physiology along with various health concerns. While this is a bit didactic, it is much like the teeny-weeny yellow polka-dot bikini; it covers the important parts, but makes no pretense about covering everything. I usually make no great attempt to remember statistics anyway. The descriptions and statements that follow are my own interpretations and will serve the purpose of giving a general and relatively simple background. I readily admit that I love to kick up my feet and tell stories, so here goes.

What is "old" or "elderly" anyway? Some folks, particularly those who aren't there yet, will rear back and opine robustly that it is a state of mind. Well, that's only partially correct. What I really don't understand is how my thoughts seem to remain somewhere in my thirties or forties in spite of the fact that my creaky and achy body tells me otherwise. I've seen many people who are "old" at age fifty when we become eligible for the AARP draft. Then again, I've run across some individuals who are vigorous and active in their seventies, eighties, and nineties, even to the extent of riding a motorcycle, flying a plane, or bicycling in France with a new wife. I know a flight instructor who is still working in his eighties and plenty sharp, too. I want to be like that when I grow up. It's not all genetic either. Not by a long shot.

Life expectancy in the United States is now calculated at seventy-eight for men and eighty-one for women. If you've reached three score and ten and are reading this, it's likely to be a good deal longer—even into the nineties. For lots of reasons, including smoking, obesity, diabetes, and high blood pressure, reaching seventy is more of an obstacle course for some of us.

In the matter of genetics, I would have to consider myself very fortunate. Both sets of grandparents were well into their eighties when they died. Actually, my paternal granddad was ninety-six. He was a farmer in the days when farming meant real manual labor. Although he was known to be a ladies' man in younger days, he never smoked or chewed tobacco. He never drank coffee or tea, and I doubt if he ever weighed more than 140 pounds. Extremely modest in his use of alcohol, he would take an occasional sweetened dram to be sociable. He plowed with a pair of huge draft horses, Doll and Prince, until he was seventy-six. After one of them crowded him in the stall, breaking a couple of ribs, that was it; he sold them.

My maternal grandfather presented an excellent study in the opposite direction. A big guy, a square-headed German type, not grossly obese, he was strong and muscular and could outwrestle his three boys when he was in his sixties. He did hard physical farm labor as a young man, but starting in midlife he became sedentary. Never a drinker (to my knowledge), he was a lifelong smoker. Though he lived to be eighty-six, in his final years he suffered from dementia, diabetes, and was minus both legs—amputated because of vascular disease. I've often wondered how long he might have lived in reasonable health if he had kept his weight down, stayed active, and never smoked.

I remember both my grandmothers as being somewhat fluffy and very huggable. Both of them died in their mid-eighties. I don't remember any particular health problems with them other than being overweight. Back in those days, older people's health concerns weren't considered to be an appropriate concern for children, or "chaps," as we were sometimes called. I do remember them as wonderful cooks. I loved their biscuits and jelly, as well as their chicken and dumplings, and ambrosia fruit bowls.

In the good old US of A we've been raised for the last seventy or so years to expect that we would be somewhat taken care of in our later years if we worked hard and contributed to Social Security. I can't help but contrast this to the ways of the Plains Indian tribes in dealing with their elders who became infirm and unable to travel. They were taken off to a remote place with food and water for a few days or even left in camp while the rest of the tribe migrated to other quarters. I'm sure that other aboriginal societies had similar customs. Simply explained, food, shelter, and clothing were in short supply, always, and the society was unable to support nonproductive members. It does seem cruel, though, doesn't it?

Somewhere in my readings from the distant past I remember a science-fiction tale about an all-seeing, all-knowing, controlling machine (computer-based, no doubt) that required all individuals to be tested periodically. The machine would then supply needed medication or treatment of all illness. When an individual became unproductive, the machine would administer the proper dose of a slow poison. Voilà—problem solved!

In that scenario, the people were manipulated mechanically and automatically. We're fortunate in having a government to which we may turn for care, if needed. Isn't it nice that we're still able to vote and have effective lobbyists on our behalf? My understanding, gathered from various sources and commentators, is that the Social Security program is fiscally sound and will remain so. Certainly the program will require tweaking and modifications but it remains as sound as our country and will be there to provide care, comfort, and support to those of us who are older or become infirm.

Of course there will continue to be those prophets of doom and disaster who seek fame and fortune by titillating our worst fears.

I will state, again, after a lot of this meandering, that I can't be comprehensive in the presentations I make in this book. There are way too many nooks and crannies involved. I will admit to having fun in relating all the stuff to you. This is certainly one aspect of medical practice that I have missed since my retirement more than a decade ago. Again, there are many sources, especially in this age of the Internet that can be tapped for more detailed information.

Chapter 1:

Appearance and Self-Respect

Narcissism seems to be a rare occurrence in us older folks. This isn't to say that we have little or no concern about how we look. Really, I haven't known many whom I suspect of spending an excessive amount of time in front of a mirror, adjusting this or that or admiring what they see. Well, perhaps one of my brothers. If we do spend time there we are likely working frantically to repair the time-ravaged features that stare back at us. Witness our partially bald brethren who carefully arrange those last long wisps to cover that shining pate in some fashion. To be fair, we men don't have our shelves as full of creams and lotions all guaranteed to plump out skin and cover wrinkles and the various spots and blemishes of advancing years as do our female counterparts. Cosmetic marketing is headed in that direction, though. And, of course they really hit the gray hair and balding bit.

Weight

So, sure, we do care about how we look. If the least touch of vanity isn't there, someone needs to be thinking about depression or dementia. Thus far, I have avoided the elephant in the room. That's me, of course, with many extra pounds that are responding to the call of gravity more than I would like. There is scant comfort in "fat is where it's at," "pleasingly plump," "portly," "generous," "substantial," "prosperous," and all those other euphemisms. There are many reasons for maintaining an appropriate body weight, of which appearance may be the least important. We will pick up the health implications of obesity in another chapter.

Posture

Speaking of gravity, look at the posture of some of your older buddies. Don't they seem to be shrinking to you? Slumping? Shoulders down and forward, back rounded out? Well, some of this is osteoporosis, but a lot isn't. We do tend to shrink in height, at least, with advancing years. This is due to a settling, the degeneration of connective tissue and advancing curvature of the spine. Personally, I have lost almost two inches in height since youth. Muscle weakness is involved also, and, yes, as we age, again, we want to surrender to gravity.

If you have ever been involved in acting on stage, you learn that one aspect of a character is posture. Another is movement. Younger people are more likely to stride and to stand erect with shoulders back. Age brings on a tendency to take smaller, wider steps and to slump when one stands or sits. I find myself beginning to shuffle sometimes, which seems easier, but makes you appear more weak and vulnerable. I have to remind myself to stride and walk in a confident manner. Try this. You will take years off of your appearance.

Clothing

Clothing may not tell all about us, but it does say a lot. If your clothes are clean, reasonably arranged, and appropriate for the season, you're unlikely to be seen as confused, disoriented, or possibly demented. In fact, when you do see an older male with food stains down his shirt front, urine stains on his pants, disheveled clothing, a belt that has forgotten his waist, hair sprouting from his nose and ears, hair on his head unkempt, with body odor emanating from several sources, you're looking at someone who is depressed, demented, or half-blind—maybe all of the above. Of course,

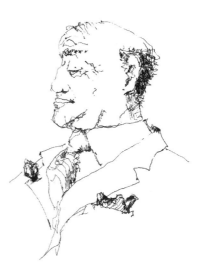

this isn't just confined to us old farts. It's a problem with older women as well (old fartresses?). No matter which sex, it's a sad situation and at that point, a care situation exists.

We men seem to find more colorful clothing to wear as we age. Sometimes I wonder why, but hey, what's wrong with that? We've worn dark pinstripes and gray this and that for far too long. Historically, the males have been among the most elaborate and colorful dressers. This cor-

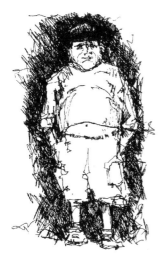

responds to the animal kingdom, particularly birds, where the males use their naturally more colorful plumage to attract their mates. There's nothing wrong with being impeccably dressed, or, for that matter, just neatly dressed. Women love a uniform or a tuxedo, and it's a foolish male who doesn't think a little about the female as he dresses. I like to take my wife with me when I shop for clothes. I definitely want her to like how I look. Most of us need all the help we can get!

3

Do deliver me, though, from ancient and torn jeans, tattoos, and dressing as your grandchildren might. You really don't look younger or hip with this stuff—just foolish. There's still a lot to be said for comfort, though. Most of our casual attire doesn't begin to feel good until it's beginning to fall apart.

One other thing: Don't even think about thongs on overweight and aging bodies at the pool or beach. Not a pretty sight on man or beast!

Chapter 11

Wellness and, on the Flip Side, Illness

"Santé!" the French say as they tip a glass of wine. "To your health!" Indeed, that wish is a reality when one considers that moderate alcohol intake, particularly wine, is good for health. Maintaining good health is one of the greatest concerns we have as the years rush by us.

We old farts don't like to think of ourselves as sick or ill. We have that macho "bull of the woods" mentality that

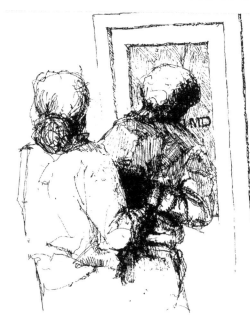

tries to tell us that it ain't going to happen to us. Ridiculous, of course. We're just as liable as the female side of the equation to get sick. Women, due to the necessity of getting medical care for pregnancy and childbirth, are much more likely to seek medical care for health problems before they become serious. Another way of looking at it: There isn't a damn thing protective about testosterone. The male of the species being more aggressive and adventuresome is more likely to get injured or to die accidentally. At any rate, we don't tolerate disability very well. It's interesting, though. Some of us get huffy and want to refuse care, while others of us regress into the dependency of childhood rather easily.

Two very important things that all of us can do for our health:

1. Accept responsibility for it.
2. Be proactive about it.

Medical Care

Medical care does little good for the individual who will not turn a hand to help himself. Exercise! Maintain proper weight! Quit smoking! Make sure you have regular medical evaluations to identify health issues before they become chronic and have complications. Diabetes, hypertension, chronic lung disease, arteriosclerosis in all its various forms, these and even cancer are much less threatening, even subject to cure, when found early. I say this especially to those individuals who fear getting health evaluations because they're afraid of finding out that they have a serious problem. I will also say it to those who have an unreasonable dread of a procedure such as a colonoscopy. Similarly, some of us even hide symptoms or go into self-denial until it's too late.

I well remember the seventy-year-old sweet little lady who presented in the office one day with rather advanced breast cancer erupting through the skin. She was so afraid that she would lose the breast that she put it off and put it off until she lost her life.

Accidents

Accidents are the leading cause of disability and death as we get older. Some of the reasons for this are: progressive weakness of those muscles that stabilize us, loss of ability to balance (caused by middle-ear problems and lack of exercise), the drop in blood pressure that can occur as our arteries stiffen (atherosclerosis), temporary decrease in blood supply to the brain (TIA), and minor strokes. The resulting falls can cause anything from bruises and minor fractures to broken hips and fatal hemorrhage into the head. With prompt treatment and care, the results can be encouraging. If the victim is alone and has no ability to communicate the distress, hours may pass without help and serious delays, prolonged recovery, and even death may ensue. In this instance, a cell phone or some other device can be lifesaving, but you have to carry it on your person!

Taking Care of Yourself

I have to say this about the subject of personal health and welfare. There is no way that anyone will care more about your well-being than you can. No one, even all the king's horses and all the king's men, can protect you or heal you if you aren't willing to take personal responsibility in these efforts. Sure, your significant other is going to have great concern about your health. He or she also ought to be concerned about whether or not your life insurance policy is up to date and paid. And this is not to say that the field of medicine can't be of some help, even in the face of your personal neglect. But the salient fact remains that your personal efforts to stop smoking, exercise, avoid or correct obesity, and be moderate in your alcohol intake will do as much if not more than the medications you take toward giving you a healthy, long life.

It's certainly good to have a companion with you if you're getting weaker and having more difficulty moving around. Giving up precious independence is, after all, a small price to pay for your security. If you have a care-giver, cherish him or her. Use a cane or walker, use hand-rails in the bathroom, and have your home surveyed for awkward areas and traps. Beware of small scatter rugs. Try to avoid those heavily advertised mobility scooters and booster chairs; their use will make you weaker, in my opin-ion. You can't save muscle strength; you only gain it with use and exercise.

Again, cell phones and devices with which you can communicate for emergency care can be vital, but they should be attached to you. Consider assisted living or simi-lar housing, especially if you're alone.

Now, you will have noticed that in reality, all of this mis-sive is pretty much dedicated to wellness and to illness. Forgive me if I repeat myself, but it's hard to overempha-size some of these basic aspects of living well. Whether or not we choose to do something about it is our own affair. Sometimes I wish I had the resolve that my paternal grand-father had. He never bit into a hot potato twice. Early in the 1920s he bought a Model T Ford. These were cantan-kerous at times. Once, it quit on him while fording a creek. Now, you had to have the spark adjustment and gas it just right when you cranked the old Ford. The early models didn't have a starter. Also, you had to have your thumb on the same side of the crank as your fingers, otherwise, when it kicked back, as frequently happened, you could break your thumb. Well, on this occasion it kicked back, hit him in the mouth, and broke his upper plate. He promptly sold the Model T and never owned another car—didn't mind riding in someone else's, though. If I had that kind of grit, I would do better at modifying my eating, lose my excess weight and realize improvement in a lot of areas.

We don't rehabilitate as easily as women do either. We tend to get withdrawn and depressed, to go off and grump in the corner. The best and fastest recovery that I have seen in males is in younger athletes who are intensely motivated to get back in the game, whatever it is. I think a lot of this occurs in younger military members who are injured as well. As we get older, though, this push to get better drops off. The missing ingredients are grit and determination. I'm sure you've noticed, as I have, that those individuals who tend toward being feisty seem to live longer and are in better health. This is one case where it's the nice guys who seem to die off at a younger age. Yep, no reward here for the virtuous!

Exercise

We do have to plan to live the best quality of life with longevity. Every generation has preached moderation in all things in pursuit of this. Exercise when we're younger doesn't need to be moderate, but it does need to be consistent. Obviously, a younger person who is training for the Olympics has to push the envelope. No way can an older person continue at this level of intensity. We do see some remarkable examples, though, in people who have been able to maintain a high level of fitness as the years pass. There are so many ways that one can exercise. It's important to find something that is pleasurable. Water aerobics works well for me now. I wish I had done more hiking when my joints were young enough to perform well. Gyms and fitness programs are great, but again, one has to be persistent and consistent. A trainer is a lot of help, particularly when one has a goal or needs help in setting one. Everywhere you care to look, from popular publications to the most scientific of journals, exercise is the single most important factor in quality of life and longevity. Even a modest amount, such as walking up to two miles a day, doing thirty minutes to an hour of aerobics daily, three times a week is more beneficial to your health that almost any medication. We are talking about diseases, strokes, and heart attacks here, serious stuff that we potentially face.

Food

The flip side of this is food intake. We are in the midst of a national epidemic of obesity that extends from earliest childhood through adolescence. A fat baby is not necessarily a healthy baby. Eating is a comforting activity. The crying baby gets more food, but may only need a good burp. Kids get cookies when they fall down and skin their knees. Some of us seem to lose our appetite when in distress; others of us gorge. Remember that 3,500 calories equal one pound of weight gain when the calorie intake is over and above that which is necessary for the activities of daily living. From somewhere, I remember that average activity burns 15 calories per pound of body weight. It really isn't that hard to gain a pound a week when we're concentrating on fast food. Fats and carbohydrates are cheaper than protein. Salads are a pretty good bargain, but watch out for the dressings.

I could not begin to recommend a specific eating plan or diet, commercial or otherwise. If any of these were extremely successful, it would dominate the field and would not need to be so heavily advertised or recommended. It would be difficult, though, to overdo vegetables, fruits, and a good level of water intake while eating a good amount of protein and limiting fats and carbohydrates. One can't help but remember the good old days before so much manufactured food was available. Our grandparents and great-grandparents would sit down to a hefty meal at noontime, have a short nap, then go out and plow the south forty. Supper was light, perhaps consisting of a few leftovers, maybe corn bread and buttermilk, followed shortly by bedtime. If these folks had antibiotics and a modest amount of medical and surgical care, we would have seen a lot more centenarians out of the group.

Illness

Well, let's talk about illness a bit. Us old farts don't like or accept illness very well, as I stated above. Not only that, but we tend to put off seeking medical care when we do get ill. It's a judgment call, of course. Much of illness is a cold or minor viral infection. Please remember, though, that it's much easier to treat an illness early than it is to wait until it's well established and developing complications. Recovery is much quicker as well. And, while most of us (I think) don't want to be whining to our significant other, he or she does need to be made aware that something is not right. After all, he or she is going to be a more objective observer of our condition than we're likely to be. I heard of one family where the senior old fart apparently had a terminal cancer of some sort. He refused to give his wife or any of the children any information about this, even to the point of not allowing them to get any information from his doctor. I don't know what kind of dysfunctions this family had, but this was not a happy time.

I really do think that in almost every case it is better to share tough conditions and decisions with each other. To do otherwise can deprive all of the family of an opportunity to plan, love, and work its way through these difficult circumstances together. Obviously, there will be times when it's not possible to do this. Some illnesses such as dementia are sneaky and can make planning impossible once underway. That means the time to make plans about end-of-life health care and to decide health care power of attorney is when one is reasonably healthy and competent. I don't think it would be morbid to plan one's own funeral either. Hey, it could be one hell of a party... with you there in spirit!

Chapter III:

Exercise

I have one thing to say about exercise. I hate it, or rather; I hate the necessity of it. I've never been athletically inclined. I never cared about being a jock. I sniffed at pitching baseball in high school, but chewing tobacco gave me bad heartburn, and I wouldn't practice. Even if you've had these leanings in the past, I would say that most of us haven't been consistent about exercising or playing games after reaching adulthood. Golf would be an exception, although it's rather modest in actual exertion. Personally, I came to a realization that exercise was an essential part of life somewhere in my mid-fifties.

Here's a news flash: I just got back from a session at the gym. It's just been a week since I resumed workouts, following a prolonged holiday break. I already feel better! Maybe it's just in my head, but hey, I'll take it. Exercise is at the very core of our ongoing, healthy existence. It goes far beyond the old saw "use it or lose it." Physical activity, or the lack of it, affects every fiber of our being. Let's look at some.

Strength and coordination: Necessary for mobility, balance, driving the car, and avoiding falls and other accidents. The loss of these two can lead to confinement, becoming bedridden or even death. Mobility directly affects the quality of life. The more one sits in a chair, the sooner one is confined to that chair. This is a prime reason that I'm not a fan of these mobility scooters that are so highly touted. The less one walks, the less one can walk, and the sooner one becomes dependent on others for care.

Cardiovascular: The heart is a muscle. Our blood vessels are lined with muscle cells. Like all types of muscle, they require exercise to maintain good function. Those blood vessels, roughly a mile of them for each pound we carry (ouch!), service every bit of our bodies from toenails to scalp. Do you think more circulation and therefore more oxygen would help the brain work better? Damn right! Exercise! Want to improve skin tone? Exercise! Decrease the pain and stiffness of arthritis? Exercise! While we can't ignore hardening of the arteries, we can stave off this process and even build new circulation around blockages with just moderate exercise.

State of mind: You may have heard of a "runner's high." Achieving this requires more vigorous activity than most of us are willing to pursue, but there's still substantial benefit to our psyche from modest exertion. With active exertion we release chemicals in the brain known as endorphins and encephalins, which are hugely responsible for our feeling of well-being. When levels of these chemicals are low, we feel rundown and flat, lack energy, and are depressed. Incidentally, stimulants such as cocaine, amphetamines, and alcohol cause us to release endorphins and encephalin too quickly and in large amounts, leaving us with a deficit. On the other hand, antidepressants seem to work by building these levels up.

General health: How are you doing with your weight? Too much? Again, a pound of weight gain represents 3,500 surplus calories. Brisk walking burns approximately 400 calories per hour. Golfing without a cart burns approximately 350 calories per hour. Swimming burns 400 calories per hour. Singles tennis burns about 700 calories per hour. Jogging burns 900 calories per hour. Resistance training burns calories as well, about 500 per hour, the amount depending on the level of exertion, of course. Conditioned muscles not only function better, but they burn calories more efficiently. Immune systems become stronger. With exercise, arthritic joints gain range of motion and produce more lubrication. Cartilage is rebuilt. And it seems unnecessary to say that sexual activity improves, sometimes dramatically.

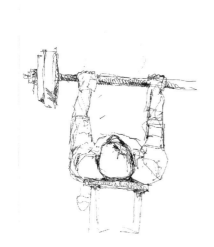

Fortunately, our bodies are in a constant state of being recycled, and, yes, it's better with exercise. Personally, I'll never enjoy working out at the gym. Some people do, and that's fine. I do like water aerobics, though. The exercise we get from sports can be a lot of fun. Be cautious and sensible though. Don't start a competitive sport in which you have no previous, continuous, experience after say, age fifty. By doing so, you're at risk for injury—perhaps serious injury. Any exercise or exertion should start gradually and build up slowly. Of course, this becomes more necessary when one is overweight or poorly conditioned and older or when one has problems such as diabetes, hypertension, and coronary artery disease. Any age or condition can benefit from exercise, but you should discuss this with your physician.

I remember a woman in her middle years who, as part of her complaint stated that her fingernails were thin and fragile and broke easily. At the time she wasn't exercising at all. She started a walking program with weight loss in mind. Several months later she casually mentioned that her fingernails were stronger and thicker. This wasn't a coincidence. The microcirculation to the nail beds had improved—with exercise. How about that? It may seem a stretch to say that every aspect of our health and our lives is better with exercise, but it's hard to think of one that isn't.

Chapter IV:

Handling Stress

Notice I haven't said anything about avoiding stress. We can't avoid it. There are many books written about avoiding stress. TV programming is awash with various experts telling us how to avoid stress. They don't really mean this. Our entire being functions with stress in every way we can imagine. We can't develop properly without the benefits of stress. It has been said that if we were to grow up in outer space without the "stress" of gravity we would develop into a circular blob. No thanks!

Physical Stress

Our muscles, bone, and connective tissue grow strong in response to the stress of gravity and the necessity of moving, carrying loads and protection. The immune system develops in large part by being challenged with the stress of infection or their manufactured substitute, vaccines. We produce red blood cells according to our body's need for oxygen. If we live at higher altitudes (thinner air, less oxygen) we produce more of them. Our brain and nervous system developed to enable us to communicate, to move in response to a threat, or, in other words, to cope with the stress and needs of daily living. As examples, humans have a large portion of their brain involving that primary sense, vision while the brain of a dog has a large portion of its substance devoted to the primary sense of smell.

OK, what happens when our bodies can't handle or adapt to stress? Think for a moment about the musculoskeletal system. Our bodies are marvelous machines. Some of us who've been privileged to dissect this miraculous body regard the study of anatomy as a near religious experience. But, nonetheless, we are machines. We have an operating life. We have load limits. Just ask those intricate structures—knees, hips, and shoulders—what happens when we overload them? They wear out faster, have a shorter service life. Ha, we're talking about arthritis, aren't we? This is the wear-and-tear kind, not that which is part of a disease such as rheumatoid, gout, or psoriatic arthritis. This isn't to say that the human mechanism can't develop compensatory ways to accommodate a different lifestyle. I think of the Masai tribe in Africa whose way of life involves running, sometimes for long distances. They would have strong cartilage and lubrication for their joints. The same is true of lifelong athletes, although there is a tendency to overstress, strain, and tear up joint mechanisms in competition.

We do have a lot of ability to self-service our bodies, to heal. One of the basic functions of any organism is to return itself to a normal state after an injury, but sometimes we need the help of a mechanic.

Mental Stress

Most of us think of stress, though, in terms of the psyche. This is really what the magazine articles and books on avoiding stress are talking about. Here again, we develop strength in response to stress. Suppose one could take an infant and protect it from emotional stress all of its childhood and developmental years. Is there anyone who believes that such an individual could function with any competence in society, particularly on his or her own? The greatest single skill our parents and families can teach us is problem solving. In fact, many, maybe most, of the difficulties we face as adults are due to an inability to deal effectively with the problems we face, to deal with the stress that is constantly present in every aspect of our lives.

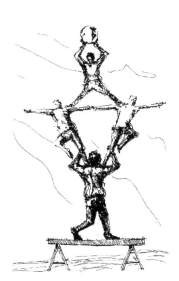

How do we gain these precious skills? Mostly from observation. And whom do we observe the most? You got it, our parents. Unfortunately, our parents may not be there for us, or they may not be all that skilled in coping themselves. Then, there's that terrible tendency some of us have to be overprotective of our children, particularly our sons. Funny, lately, I'm hearing of "helicopter parents," hovering a lot, of course. If we constantly pull our children's chips out of the fire so that they never suffer consequences for their improper actions, even as little kids, they won't develop proper coping skills. You can expect more of these individuals to have antisocial, lawbreaking, or even fatal outcomes. Of course, at the age most of you are reading this, it's too late to be of much effect on your children, but we can stick an oar in for the grandchildren.

Well, the above is certainly of interest, but here we are, older and hopefully wiser. How do we as "mature" people deal with our anxieties and our inability to cope at times? Communication is essential here. We can talk to our spouses or to friends. If the situation is more serious, don't hesitate to find a counselor. Group therapy works nicely also. For many problems, exercise can help. Remember, exercise increases those brain chemicals that have to do with feeling good. Activities of many kinds can be beneficial. Singing in a choir and community chorus works for me. Try to make medications a last resort, if possible.

Now, if depression is a significant part of the problem, medication may be needed. However one gets there, low levels of certain brain chemicals characterize depression. Remember that drugs such as alcohol, marijuana, cocaine, and amphetamines rip through these chemicals like a tornado, leaving us with a deficit, which can be profound. Any deficit is responsible for anxiety and feelings of doom and gloom together with feelings of unease and impending disaster. Suicidal thoughts can be frequent, even natural. If they do become obsessive, immediate help can be lifesaving.

Even if that's tough, try to regard stress as a learning and developmental experience. I know this sounds good, but I don't think stress will ever be regarded as a friend, unless you're a skydiver, daredevil, or some other kind of adrenaline junkie.

The Brain: Part One, How It Works

Assuming that the ancients did indeed consider the heart as a seat of the soul and the liver as the seat of the various humors that affect us, they had many different ideas and theories about the function of the brain. One of the more ancient ideas was that it was a radiator to cool the blood. Another was that it was the receptacle of the spirit and could be affected in bad ways by the entrance of evil spirits. If one puts all these different concepts together, though, the ancients had a fair idea in general of the importance of the brain and its many functions. (It's hard to buy the concept of a radiator for the blood, however.) Attempts to further define brain function continued through the Middle Ages and Renaissance and into recent times. This organ is the command center of the entire organism. All creatures have some rudiments of a brain, at least. Those of us who possess some semblance of thought are blessed—or possibly cursed—with a good deal more development in the brain.

The more basic critters, above the simplest organisms, have a brain stem wherein the vegetative functions such as breathing, heart rate, temperature control, balance, sleep, blood pressure, alertness, and other housekeeping functions are regulated.

The cerebellum is concerned with our motor activity, particularly fine movement and coordination. The cerebral cortex is responsible for the vast number of activities that are concerned with the development of higher organisms. The frontal lobe deals with our emotional responses, judgment, expressive language, memory of habits, and some motor function. The parietal lobes have to do with manipulation of objects, multitasking, integration, touch, perception, and visual attention. The occipital lobes are almost entirely devoted to vision. The temporal lobes are devoted to hearing, memory, and have some activity in the visual realm and for organization. The brain contains somewhere in the neighborhood of 100 billion neurons, and there are zillions of interconnections between these neurons. Computers have a long way to go.

When I was in medical school, there were a half dozen or so brain chemicals known to us. At present there are thousands, with more being described all along. We used to think that much of the brain was unused or at least poorly used. It was fun to speculate what we would be like if we were able to use most or all of our brain functions. Current thinking is that we do indeed use a great deal more of the brain than we thought we did. Further, we know that there is an incredible amount of interconnectivity and switching activity that goes on among the areas of the brain.

Memory is one of the prime attributes of higher brain function. Most of us are aware that dogs have an olfactory sense that is thousands of times more sensitive to smell than that of humans. As I stated before, much of the canine brain is devoted to the memory of odors. This general principle applies to all organisms. We develop what we need to survive, reproduce, and become more efficient. An easy example: The blind individual develops more brain activity related to hearing and touch.

The brain is, of course, divided into two hemispheres, and it's interesting that they're not duplicates. Most of us are right-handed, and the left side of the brain has more control functions than the right. Under some circumstances, we can function with half a brain. This has been shown to be the case particularly in young individuals who've had half the brain removed because of intractable seizures or malignancy. The right brain seems to have more to do with artistic and creative pursuits and is sometimes thought to be the more feminine side of the brain. Left-handed individuals are sort of a curiosity. Their brains, at least, seem to be hooked up backward to some degree. It's also been proven that left-handed individuals are more capable of using both sides of the brain. This is probably the result of our civilization pushing the left-handers toward usually right-handed activities. It's been shown that left-handers survive strokes and retain function more easily than do righties.

As you might suspect, the brain, being in control, gets first crack at the oxygenated blood leaving the heart. The left and right carotid arteries in the neck are large and travel up the sides of the neck, just under the ear, before going through the skull and entering the cerebral circulation. The brain is also a heavy user of energy. We supply this energy to the brain in the form of a simple sugar, glucose. This doesn't mean that you can throw more coal in the furnace (glucose) and get more heat, or brain activity. It could be a reason, though, for hyperactivity in kids that eat a lot of carbohydrates.

Stroke

If the supply of oxygen and energy to brain cells is interrupted longer than four minutes, brain cells start dying off. This is the critical reason for prompt efforts at resuscitation. More recently, there have been efforts to dissolve blood clots that have blocked a portion of the cerebral circulation. More efficient diagnostic work has been done to determine whether a stroke is due to hemorrhage or to a clot. Emergency personnel certainly don't want to be in the position of making hemorrhage worse by adding anticoagulants. Blood clots, usually from calcium plaques that have developed in the arterial circulation, are the most common cause of stroke. They are silent, painless, and can strike at any time, but frequently do so during the night or early morning hours. These can be massive and fatal (not a bad way to go really), or so minor as to be almost undetectable. These can be a wicked cause of progressive dementia, and I've always likened the multiple-small-stroke syndrome to watching the lights go out in a house with lighted windows at night. The degree of function lost following a stroke is entirely due to the amount of brain tissue lost. People worry about running their blood pressure up to a high level and causing a stroke. This would be rare, and the blood pressure would have to be at an extraordinarily high level. It's the chronic, long-term blood pressure elevations that predispose to thickening in the arterial blood vessels and more frequent strokes.

The kind of stroke that really will get your attention is due to hemorrhage. It's usually caused by the rupture of a small, balloon-like defect in the small arteries at the base of the brain. These aneurysms are associated with heredity. Being at the base of the brain, they're very difficult to approach surgically and are frequently fatal. The pain is of sudden onset and usually described as "the worst headache I've ever had." Sometimes it's accompanied by a stiff neck and is always a subject for emergency intervention. The loss of brain cells in these cases is usually due to the increasing pressure of the hemorrhage.

Head trauma is a fairly frequent cause of hemorrhage within the skull. While this can happen at any age, our arterial blood vessels become more rigid and lose flexibility as we age. Sometimes even a minor fall or blow to the head can cause them to rupture and bleed extensively. I remember one older guy who lost his footing while rolling a wheelbarrow of dirt. His head hit a pile of dirt, which was relatively soft, but he still developed major hemorrhage. These hemorrhages are usually subdural, which means beneath the outer covering of the brain, and again the loss of function is due to pressure. This is not necessarily fatal or permanent, and with relief of the pressure frequently function returns. These hemorrhages can be sneaky, sometimes indicated by a slowing of thought or speech or increasing drowsiness. Incidentally, it's not dangerous to go to sleep after an injury. This bit of folklore has come about because drowsiness has long been known as a symptom. However, difficulty awakening can be a symptom also.

Trauma

The most frequent trauma in our society today is due to motor vehicle accidents. Depending on the circumstances and the severity of the injury, it's possible to have bleeding within the brain tissue itself. If one is struck by the vehicle or thrown from a vehicle, a broken neck with injury to the spinal cord is quite likely. I remember the frequent head, facial, and other severe injuries in the pre-seat-belt era, and indeed the wonderful decrease in the severity of the injuries following introduction of the airbag. I just today read of the death of two older individuals ejected from their vehicle because they weren't wearing seat belts.

Although I can't begin to cover everything in this chapter, it's difficult to leave the subject without touching on tumors and cancer within the brain. Tumor is a generic term, which simply describes a growth or swelling, which may be malignant. By definition, cancer is a growth of tissue out of its normal bounds and interwoven with the adjoining material. A simple tumor usually has a membrane or capsule around it and isn't invasive. Its effect is that of increasing pressure and size, sometimes over many years. Most cancers of the brain are metastatic. That is to say that they originate in some other organ—frequently the lungs—and are borne by the blood or lymph system to another site. Although metastasis itself is an alarming event, these tumors are easier to treat in the brain than most primary brain cancer. Some of these are notoriously resistant to therapy or surgery, but there does seem to be some recent advances that may offer hope.

Chapter V:

The Brain; Part Two
Keeping It Working

I outlined the very complex structure of the brain in the previous section. Now, it's worthwhile to think a little more about how things work. We have billions of neurons and zillions of connections. No way can we engage in a detailed analysis of brain function here, even if I knew it all, but we will talk about some of the more salient concerns.

"I don't mind getting older, if I can just keep my wits about me." That is an earnest plea that we hear all the time, and in no way is it unreasonable. The other side of that, of course, is if we lose our wits, it would be good to lose so little that it didn't make a damn bit of difference, or that we would lose enough that we couldn't appreciate what was going on anyway. We do lose some mental abilities with advancing years, but this is quite variable. Perhaps the best indicator for maintaining one's mental faculty is one over which we have absolutely no control. That is genetic. I hope that your parents and grandparents were able to maintain a good level of mental acuity throughout their life span. If they didn't fare that well, don't despair—there are ways to help preserve, even improve, what you have now.

Over the years, it's been obvious to me that school-teachers and librarians do better than most in hanging on to their smarts. This is certainly borne out in research studies. Obviously, using one's mind develops more and better brain function and slows down or compensates for a net loss of neurons. As we see from observing people who recover from strokes, the brain is capable of developing alternate pathways and repairing damage. And, there are ways to stave off, or at least slow down, the loss of brain function. Physical exercise, even modest, is one of the best. As I mentioned before, physical activity improves the circulation. This improvement isn't limited to the muscles; we require good circulation to carry oxygen and glucose to the brain and remove byproducts of metabolism. You'll think better, solve problems better, and likely have a better frame of mind with physical exercise. Again, an hour three times a week or thirty minutes daily is achievable by all of us—you don't have to be a marathon runner.

Mental exercise is just as is essential as the physical variety. For years, I've told my contemporaries, "If you're not learning, you're dying." I really believe this! Scientific studies show that the brain is stimulated to grow new neurons and pathways when challenged to learn. By now, many of us have heard the tale of cabbies in London who are required to study the streets, intersections, and byways of that very complex city before receiving their license. This takes two to four years. They actually develop a larger hippocampus (a portion of the brain that serves memory and switching functions) than the rest of us would normally have.

So now is the time for you to delve more deeply into an old interest or to develop a new one. Learn to paint. Learn music. Learn a new language. Read more. Take courses that are available at your local university or community college. Get the degree you never completed. There are academic courses available in several recorded formats by outstanding teachers in their field.

Why is it that distant memories are so much more accessible at times than our recent memories? I think I read about that somewhere recently, but—ha!—I don't remember just

WILLIAM B. WADDELL, MD

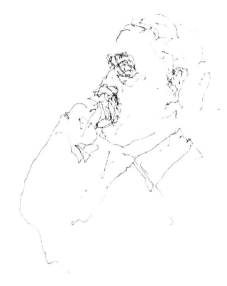

where. I've heard it said that perhaps our "in-box" gets overstuffed with so much current input that some of it falls out before it can be sorted, processed, and put into long-term memory. We enjoy thinking about times past, old ties, childhood, family, old friends. I recognize the urge to contact these friends from the past, reconnect, and find out what they've been doing. Curious, isn't it? Perhaps it's a realization of our own mortality.

Then, on the other hand, we have trouble remembering recent events, names, the answer to a question that someone has. We don't recall the answer at the moment, but we wake up with it at three in the morning. Or we wander into another room on a mission and forget what the mission was. There are mnemonic devices we can use to help recent memory. Some of us will keep logs or journals—just don't misplace them. It really is a good idea to keep family phone numbers and addresses in your wallet in case of an incapacitating accident or illness. Finally, there's no better subject for "use it or lose it" than the mind. Now *that* is a principle worth engraving on the inside of your skull!

The degree to which the mind influences the physical activities of the body is humbling. I'm not talking about feeling good or bad here, I'm talking about actual physical happenings. We all know that a positive attitude influences recovery from illness or injury. Recently, a study seemed to show that some women could have heart attacks in spite of **normal coronary arteries**.

A couple of years ago, I started having episodes of left-chest discomfort. It started when I was working as a volunteer on a construction project for one of our local organizations. It was a very hot day. I was doing strenuous work involving a nail gun. I have coronary artery disease, having had a minor attack some ten years ago. I also take blood pressure medication and cholesterol medication, and I'm overweight and well into the age when these things are relatively common.

You're probably thinking it wasn't too bright of me to be doing this. You're right. But anyway...Even though the pain was not too bad, it certainly got my attention. I went to our EMT squad, they did an EKG (no change from previous ones), I had a whiff of nitroglycerin, and the discomfort went away. Over the next two months, similar, milder episodes occurred, especially when I was a little frustrated, say, as when hurrying through an airport terminal to get to the next gate while carrying luggage. I found myself slowing down, avoiding heavier loads, and giving in to the perceived limitations of heart function. My outlook became somewhat depressed and my sense of mortality more acute. I stopped exercising, of course. My wife was concerned and tried to relieve the activities of daily living by carrying heavy groceries and luggage and bringing the car around from the parking lot. After a few weeks, I had convinced myself that I had major coronary disease, probable near blockages. Something had to be done!

At this point, you probably sense what's coming. Let me tell you, as an aside, that your run-of-the-mill hypochondriac can't hold a candle to the physician who is aware of all the possibilities and has these tendencies. Man, they aren't in the same league! I am sure there are studies on the incidence of hypochondriasis in physicians. I haven't seen one, but I'll bet it's high. To be fair to myself, I was having chest discomfort that had a classic onset and I did know that it would be foolish to try to ignore it.

My primary care physician, a very good general internist, referred me back to the cardiologist. A nuclear stress test showed, or seemed to show, a decrease in heart muscle function in the posterior and inferior cardiac wall. There was an increase in blood pressure during the test, and this persisted for a while afterward. These were somewhat ominous signs. Cardiac catheterization was indicated. This is the definitive test, wherein a radiopaque contrast medium is injected throughout the coronary arteries. At the same time, narrowed vessels can be stretched, soft blockages can be removed, and a wire coil (stent) placed if needed. Obviously it's a rather technical procedure requiring a skilled team and cardiologist. I was eager to get this done and start feeling better.

Well, we were all surprised and somewhat taken aback when no narrowed places were found. The coronary arteries were a bit ratty and had plaques consistent with my age, but the circulation was good. The chest discomfort was not coming from the heart. Whatever the origin, the problem didn't appear to be threatening or serious. I had had a reprieve! I could've danced had I not been told to take it easy for a few days to let the catheter site heal.

The next day, I was embarrassed by the ease with which I climbed the stairs. I had laboriously and slowly pulled myself up the day before. My outlook was sunnier. I felt twenty pounds lighter. Exercise, weight loss, and happier times were ahead! Now, I've known the power of mind over body all through my professional life, but never as so powerful a concept about myself and driven home so well. Clearly, the mind is a wonderful thing, but what Alcoholics Anonymous calls "stinkin' thinkin'" in another context can put us in a world of trouble.

Dementia

Dementia is sad. There seems to be more of it lately. I don't know whether this is a function of our increasing population, better diagnosis, pollution, or a longer life span. It certainly isn't a new problem. Elderly grandparents used to sit by the

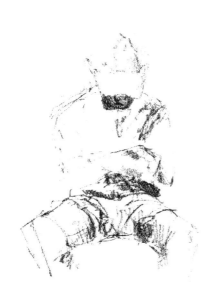

fire, smoke, and rock themselves into oblivion. This was in the homes of their children or grandchildren, and wasn't very visible to society at large and was even expected. In this day of long-term care facilities, it's certainly more obvious. There are several causes.

Alzheimer's dementia is still a pathology diagnosis. That is to say that it requires a microscopic examination of actual tissue. Not many of us are up for a brain biopsy, so the definitive diagnosis is made postmortem. This seems to be due to the accumulation of an amyloidal protein among the brain cells, and there is still disagreement as to the cause. Medications are only of modest help. Another cause of dementia is that of multiple small infarcts (blockages) in the smaller arteries supplying the brain. As stated in the section on brain anatomy, its progression is similar to watching the lights go out in a well-lit home. There are chemical causes due to various poisons. The most common of these is due to chronic alcohol abuse, and usually happens over a long period of time. There are acute forms as well. Methanol or wood alcohol poisoning used to be more common than it is now. Severely addicted persons will drink or sniff almost anything that gives an effect similar to ethyl alcohol, including the fuel, Sterno. Sniffing gasoline and other inhalant hydrocarbons can be bad, as can chronic exposure to some industrial substances. Advanced liver disease with rising ammonia levels can do a number on the brain. And there are genetic disorders such as Parkinson's disease, Huntington's chorea, and many others. Finally, there are several other diseases that produce chemical imbalance within the body that can cause dementia.

Other than those temporary, reversible, and sometimes treatable causes of dementia, the care of dementia sufferers is pretty much the same. Depending on the degree of damage and on the speed with which the disease progresses, a lot of personal care is required. Social interaction is very important. Obviously, that which can occur within the family is best, but many times this has to be done in an institution. We all know of devoted couples where one partner is afflicted. The other is committed to ongoing personal care, insofar as is possible. This is wonderful when it can happen, but frequently the unaffected partner is elderly or incapacitated in some other way also. Families are split up and widely separated and can't help.

Perhaps the unkindest cut of all is the slow-onset form of dementia, wherein the person involved is aware of the

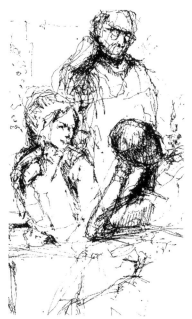

disease. Although present medications don't seem to be all that helpful, this is one place that they should certainly be tried. Of course, to do this one needs a diagnosis, if possible. The far side of dementia, at least, puts one in the condition of not being able to appreciate the degree of trouble he or she is dealing with. The family can be in a great deal of distress because they are no longer recognized due to the tremendous confusion of their loved one.

I must say again and again that exercise—both mental and physical—is the best means of holding off or even preventing the onset of dementia. There is a great deal of research going on in hopes of finding medications for this disease, but I don't think I would hold my breath.

Chapter VI:

Kinesiology 101

As a medical student, I had limited appreciation for this study of the science of movement. That came to me gradually over years of medical practice and then hit me with a thud as I entered the older years myself. It's as I've said before, our bodies are marvelous machines, truly marvelous. But, as has been appreciated from the dawn of civilization, our life span is limited. In the cosmic order of things, it's a flea flicker. How's that statement for an ego buster?

The musculoskeletal system defines the basic structure of the body, of course. Its growth follows genetic factors as well as environmental stress. Nutrition is very important. It's very interesting to me that as a group our society seems to be developing larger and taller individuals. I'm not talking about obesity. Presumably a lot of this is due to better nutrition. This is demonstrably different when a country develops better standards of nutrition for its citizens. I personally remember smaller basketball and football players sixty years ago.

Like everything else in the body, bones and muscles are in a constant state of change and require the raw materials with which to do this. The body is programmed to return to a normal state following injury. Therefore, we heal cuts and muscle tears with scar tissue and repair bone fractures with new bone formation. For example, if you break an arm or leg, it will attempt to heal without being set in normal alignment, but you may end up with a crooked arm or leg or a nonfunctioning joint. Similarly, we can heal severe cuts and injuries with bad scars, but we do much better if an attempt is made to restore the normal function and appearance. Incidentally, this has been a function of medical practitioners for many thousands of years.

Back

Homo sapiens are cursed with back trouble. Having evolved from a four-legged past, our spine has yet to fully accommodate to a vertical posture and gait. Our best bet, then, is to strengthen what we can. We might think that the spine carries the weight of the upper torso and head, but the abdominal muscles support 40 percent of the upper body. I think we could give at least 20 percent to the back muscles. This leaves the poor stacked-up vertebral bodies with intervening disks to do the rest. If you've developed six-pack abs and well-defined back muscles, you're unlikely to have back problems more serious than a simple contusion or sprain. Considering our tendency to weaken more rapidly as we age, it's a wonder that we aren't worse off than we are. I'm sure that earlier generations requiring more physical exertion for daily living had less trouble with their backs. Of course, their overall life span was shorter, due to many factors.

Muscles

Muscular strength is critical to survival in good health. Without strong legs, one is unable to balance and coordinate movement properly. Couple this with decreased sensation in the feet and lower legs that many of us develop

36

as we age and you have a scenario for unprotected falls. Although bad enough, this can be one hell of a lot more serious than, "I've fallen and I can't get up." My father died in this manner when he fell backward, striking a concrete wall while going up the stairs. He was eighty-two and had a massive head injury. I notice that I'm falling more frequently, more easily, and in a more uncoordinated fashion. So far, no serious injuries or broken bones, and I have been able to protect my head. We should not neglect upper.-torso strength either. Strong shoulder and arm muscles can modify or prevent falls as well. A good grip can be a lot of protection.

Be More Cautious

Most serious injuries to us old farts occur in and around the home. Of course, that's where we are most of the time. We're more at risk when we venture out into a world of irregular sidewalks, street curbing, traffic, or unfamiliar surroundings. I suspect that we have an increased awareness at these times and thereby don't get injured as much.

We do go downhill with advancing age and the slope gets steeper unless we do something to slow it down. Our entire system is affected, some individuals more, others less. Good genes are nice to have, though. Generally speaking, most functions slow as we age. We have less energy and it doesn't last as long as it once did. Muscular strength diminishes. The latest figures I've seen indicate a 2 percent loss of muscle strength each year after age fifty. Ouch! The sense of balance is affected, part of that being muscle loss. Brain function slows somewhat, but is compensated for, in part, by a surplus of brain cells and by experience. Reaction time is increased to the detriment of our driving skills. Bowel function slows. Sexual arousal takes longer (more about this later). Visual acuity diminishes. Hearing becomes impaired. Bones lose calcium

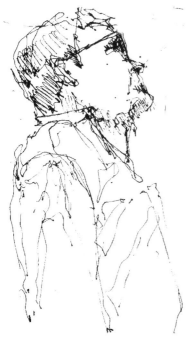

and become softer. Wear and tear on joints shows up as loss of cartilage. Our bodies stiffen everywhere but where stiffness is needed. The litany goes on and on. Much of health care is devoted to correcting or at least improving these ravages, but, individually, we still can do a lot to help ourselves. Actually, we can do more to help ourselves than the best-intentioned health care giver.

Posture and Attitude

We discussed this in the chapter about appearance and self-respect, but it's worth repeating: Your posture and the way you move go a long way toward how other people perceive us. Remember the straight-backed military posture? How about the dejected slump of the down-and-out person? Then there's the careless, spine-sitting slump of the adolescent. Think of the movement and stride of the fit and alert person. Want to set yourself up for a mugging in the city? Just mope along, shoulders down, looking vulnerable and it might happen. It's not always possible to walk with a positive stride, although exercise and practice, along with proper weight, helps to maintain this. It's really easier to stand and balance with an erect posture than it is to slump and give in to gravity. Another pearl, if we act as though we feel good, we'll feel better.

One of the tough things about degenerative diseases such as Parkinson's is some loss of the ability for facial expression. It's difficult to appear to be interested in the discussion under the circumstances. An attitude of alertness and interest conveys the impression of a younger person, or at least of someone who is older but retains an awareness of the environment he or she is in.

Activity

Bed rest and other inactivity—most notably nowadays sitting on our butts and watching television—weaken the body at any age. Again, the loss is more rapid as we get older. Activity of any sort and exercise of any kind are most important to our well-being. Even small amounts of activity are helpful. If walking is difficult, try water aerobics or other low-weight-bearing exercises.

Mobility

As an aside, I can't help but shudder when I see TV ads for booster chairs that help one stand and for motorized chair scooters that "improve mobility." Again, I hate the use of these powered scooters and mobile chairs that are being so heavily advertised. I have nothing against the use of these devices or wheelchairs when one is paralyzed in the legs or otherwise unable to walk. If you have any ability to move around using your own legs, I can almost guarantee that you will lose it if you default to a motorized device. Apparently, Medicare, Medicaid, and some insurance companies pay for these devices if a medical doctor is willing to state that ambulation is difficult. Unfortunately, it doesn't seem to be that hard to find a doctor who will state this. These things are expensive and are an incredible drain on the health care dollar. Third party payors have become more aware of this. Hopefully, we will see regulations tightened to a considerable degree on these and other health care appliances. I should be careful here; I'm getting close to a rant. Even if you have limited mobility, you're much better off using what you have and improving it. Once you commit to a motorized chair your walking days are over, in my opinion.

Devices that *assist* mobility, on the other hand, can be quite helpful. I don't like to use a cane any more than you do, but they sure are a help on uneven ground or on a long walk. Of course, they can be carried and swung in a rather debonair manner as well. A couple of generations ago, any gentlemen strolling along the boulevard would carry one. As has been said, a cane is sometimes useful for protecting one's self from those hordes of adoring females. Depending on the circumstances, three- or four-legged canes or walkers are very helpful, whether temporary or not. If you've had a knee or hip replacement done, you know what I mean. (By the way, it's not my place here to advise for or against any replacement. I've heard it said that if you can go into a squat and stand up without a good deal of pain or assistance, you do not need a replacement. Get a referral to an orthopedist that your physician feels comfortable with and go from there.)

Arthritis

"Where's the Queen?" cried the King.
"In bed with Arthritis," was the reply.
"Well, kill the Greek rascal and bring her forth!"
Isn't it odd that such snippets of memory stay with us? Small-joint arthritis can be immune malfunction (rheumatoid) or osteoarthritis (wear and tear). Moist heat, warm paraffin baths, and finally, anti-inflammatory drugs—or some combination of these—should help. Now, there are more specific drugs for rheumatoid disease. Beware of immobilization for the most part. Joints freeze up quickly, especially the shoulder. Large-joint arthritis is mostly osteoarthritis, the wear-and-tear kind. Again, like a machine, joints have a design life and deteriorate more rapidly

under excessive load. This is one reason that being over-weight is so hard on us. I used to tell my patients, "Imagine carrying twenty pounds on each shoulder every step you take, all day and every day." Ha! Now I have to tell myself that. While small-joint disease is a hallmark of rheumatoid arthritis and other inflammatory processes, be aware that there is a lot of overlap, even combinations. And, let's not forget gouty arthritis, that wonderful genetic disorder that was once considered the bane of those who overin-dulged in food and wine. At least it can be controlled by medication.

Use it or lose it! Or, as the dentist says, "If you got 'em, floss 'em"!

Chapter VII

The Ears, Eyes, and Mouth

We might as well flip down the body a ways, since we've started some physiology. We can't cover all the stuff in detail, but here goes.

Hearing

How well can you hear me now? We certainly lose acuity in hearing as we age. Much of this loss depends on the degree to which we have been exposed to noise in our environment, but there are other factors as well, such as infection and heredity. Some years ago, I had a retired Navy machinist mate working with me on projects around the house. He'd spent most of his naval career in the engine room of many vessels. As you can imagine, these are very noisy environments. He had an interesting hearing loss. He couldn't hear well in a quiet situation. When there was a lot of noise, he could hear normal conversation more easily. Practically speaking, this meant that it took a fair amount of sound energy to mobilize the mechanical aspects of the ear, and then conversational sound could be recruited on top of the noise.

As a family doctor, I occasionally extracted a full plug of wax from a patient's ear canal. The amazed looks when hearing was restored were fun to watch. Usually, we lose the higher frequencies first—just ask your wife. Aside from good social function, this can be dangerous. Recently, I was impatient and didn't insert my own hearing aids. That day, I drove up behind another car that wasn't proceeding through a green light. Still impatient, I tooted my horn. I tooted again, several times. I broke into a sweat and felt like a fool when the fire engine that I hadn't heard streaked by, sirens blasting. Hearing aids are readily available. The better and smaller ones are expensive. Do find an ethical audiologist, though, and avoid sales pitches and extravagant advertisements. One other anecdote: A few months ago my wife was telling me about this grumpy older guy that she occasionally sat close to while taking the ferry to work. He didn't seem to be interested in conversation, but was constantly reading. His social outlook totally changed though, when his wife insisted that he get hearing aids. He became more gregarious and conversational. One can't help but wonder how many of us old farts become socially isolated because of hearing loss. Sometimes we're not even aware of this.

Vision

We have more areas of the brain associated with or devoted to vision than any other sense. This immediately tells us how important our eyes are. Regular checkups as part of a physical or by an eye specialist are quite necessary. These should always include an intraocular pressure test for glaucoma. This is a simple thing to do, painless, and provides early detection for an insidious disease that can result in a total blindness.

Visual acuity changes as we age, of course. Most of us are going to need some degree of magnification to read easily. It's interesting that distant vision sometimes improves with aging. This a structural change. It's perfectly all right to buy your reading glasses over the counter. Just be sure that you're getting regular checkups and nothing else is going on.Of course, the cheaper glasses are not as consistent in quality.

Other than glaucoma, there are several other degenerative diseases that damage the vision. Retinal and macular degeneration are high on the list. Treatment for this is not yet perfect, but it's helpful. Retinal hemorrhage, prevalent in those who have diabetes and severe hypertension, is progressive, but can be treated with laser therapy. Retinal separation is an acute event, a substantial disturbance of vision, and is a bona fide emergency. The earlier treatment is accomplished, the better the result. There are a few infections that can damage the cornea, the clear visual window in front of the eye. These are usually apparent and treatable.

Some of the most satisfying results are obtained in the treatment of cataracts. Cataracts involve progressive clouding of the lens located in the front of the eye behind the iris. Before corrective glasses were invented, practitioners would displace the lens in cases of total blindness, providing at least some kind of vision. Nowadays, the lens is destroyed (emulsified), removed, and an artificial lens inserted. The same muscles used by the natural lens can focus some of these plastic lenses. Having had this done in both eyes, I can testify that it's a blast to finally do without glasses and to appreciate normal color without a yellow cast. Of course, one wants a skilled ophthalmologic surgeon who has done a number of these procedures.

Teeth

Although I don't know a lot about the technical aspects of dentistry, I have had quite a lot of dental care over the years. I do know that dental health is extremely important to overall health and well-being. Nowadays, because of advances in dentistry and dental care and hygiene, we are much better at retaining our teeth. Years ago, if an adult were in a state of advanced decay with gum disease, it was common to have a complete extraction and full plates put in. This was less expensive in the long run, but it sure is a poor solution with its own set of problems. One can look around and see that it's still being done.

Of course, it's much better to treat dental decay and any gum disease early, when it can be done less expensively. It's well known that dental disease can be a source of systemic infection and subsequent poor health. It's a lot less expensive to practice good dental hygiene—brushing, flossing, and so forth—from the start, hopefully avoiding more expensive treatment and not risking your health. If it's necessary, though, do whatever you need to do. Spending on dental health is well worth it. I'm assuming that you enjoy food as much as I do.

One other thought: The dentist usually checks for early cancer in the mouth and on the lips. These are much more frequent in tobacco users. Add tobacco use to heavy alcohol intake, and one begins to see more cancers of the mouth and throat, particularly with snuff or tobacco chewing.

There's probably no need to mention the social implications of bad breath. Poor dental hygiene is a major factor. There are other causes for this, such as constipation and poor dietary habits. But, halitosis beats no breath at all. For many years, I worked with a surgeon who had terrible teeth with a lot of decay and gum disease. While he did manage to control most of his bad breath, he was in the habit of talking with his hand over his mouth. His dentist finally talked him into having some restorative work, whereupon his smile and his personality dramatically improved. Some of us, like this guy, have an irrational fear of dental drilling and other techniques. Believe me, the newer, high-speed drills; advanced anesthetic; and cooling methods have taken a lot of the discomfort out of dental care. Get it done and keep it done—and, yeah, if you got 'em, floss 'em.

Chapter VIII:

The Chest, Lungs, and Breathing

We are an aerobic species. We require oxygen and exchange it with carbon dioxide in the lungs. Much of the quality and longevity of our lives have to do with the health of our respiratory system. The very air that we breathe is full of pollutants, most of it by far man-made. Have you ever wondered how ancient astronomers discovered so many of our planets and stars? Interpolating backward, scientists have determined that the atmosphere was incredibly clear in ancient times. There was much less smoke from cooking and heating. Some of these external environmental factors we can control. Much of it is due to increased population density producing polluted air, polluted water, and various toxins. We can, however, push for a cleaner, greener society.

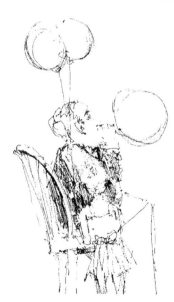

You wouldn't believe the difference in the appearance of newborn lungs and the lungs of a person past fifty, even without considering work environment. The older person's lungs are nearly black and stiff, while the infant's lungs are pink and elastic, very inflatable. It's obvious that the work environment has a great deal to do with this. The coal miner, the rock miner, and those who work in smoke and dust lose respiratory capacity earlier. Our genetic inheritance determines a lot of the speed with which this happens.

Smoking

By now, everyone knows that tobacco smoke does a number on lung tissue. All of the environmental causes noted above are greatly aggravated by tobacco smoke. I used to be amazed at the difference in lung function in miners being evaluated for black lung disease. The X-rays of smokers and nonsmokers might have looked equally bad, but the smokers had lost a great deal more of their capacity to exchange oxygen and carbon dioxide. Just recently, I read that there's been a large decrease in cancers, particularly in males, due to the decrease of smoking in the population, and that's terrific news.

Not every smoker gets lung cancer, and every person with lung cancer is not a smoker, but the statistics are frightening. Sidestream, or secondary, smoke is bad as well. In my family practice, I recall two nonsmokers, one male, one female, who died of small-cell lung cancer (the smoker's variety) from their spouse's sidestream smoke. Perhaps the worst complication from smoking is chronic bronchitis and emphysema, popularly known in TV advertisements as COPD, the abbreviation for chronic obstructive pulmonary disease. Talk about the speed with which lungs stiffen and reduce the ability to exchange—smoking puts this on wheels. Sure, all of us know people who have been smokers and don't seem to be affected all that much. One of my great-grandmothers smoked a corncob pipe and lived to an advanced age. So what! Maybe she didn't inhale.

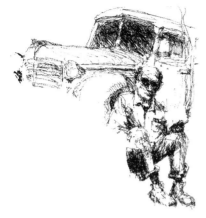

For more than forty years, I've heard people say, "I don't care if I die fifteen years earlier because I smoke. I don't want to live to be elderly and decrepit." These folks have the very mistaken idea that they will reach the end of a healthy life and suddenly drop dead. This might well happen with a sudden stroke or coronary, but think again, guys; it's much more likely that you will spend your last months or years sucking on an oxygen tube or a respirator, perhaps with a tracheotomy (that's a surgical opening in the windpipe). That isn't any way to enjoy a full and complete life.

Tobacco really is a disaster for the cardiorespiratory system. Chewing and dipping have their own set of problems. Coronary artery disease, peripheral artery disease, and atherosclerosis, in general, are all accelerated by tobacco. There are other strong factors, such as elevated cholesterol, diabetes, obesity, and genetics. All factors multiply, of course—it's not just simple addition.

Sleep Apnea

Have you ever heard of sleep apnea? There's been a lot more attention paid to this problem of late. Briefly, this can be described as an aggravated degree of snoring, to the point where the normal breathing pattern is interrupted. The individual stops breathing for up to thirty seconds or so. The sleeper partially awakens and resumes his or her usual breathing (snoring) pattern and does the same thing over and over. This happens throughout the night and is readily demonstrated in sleep studies. The blood oxygen level drops, and healthy sleep is not possible. While aging tissues in the throat are part of the problem, obesity is a big factor. It's most common in males. There's considerable reason for concern. We need normal sleep for good health.

Sleep apnea's been proven to be a factor in dementia, hypertension, heart disease, and irritated spouses. Frequently, we're made aware of this when our significant other says, "If you don't get something done about this snoring, I'm going to move to the other bedroom." I've run across some notable snorers in my day. Some of these guys could rattle the windows. Years ago, I was duck hunting with a bunch of guys. We stayed overnight in a cabin. One of the party, a dentist, was that kind of snorer. The rest of us struggled to get to sleep before he went to bed. Finally, a brave individual said, "I can fix this." He went to the dentist's room and planted a big kiss full on his mouth. Needless to say, the snorer stayed awake all night.

Now we have medical evidence that this apnea isn't healthy. I've seen this condition in a few kids with enlarged tonsils and adenoids. Surgery is indicated here and is curative. In a skinny individual with the problem, surgery can be effective.

A little bedside machine called a CPAP (computerized pressure assist pump) is a bit of a nuisance to use, but corrects the problem. You have to wear a nasal mask or pillow and keep the mouth closed to make it work. This really isn't so bad, but it takes some getting used to. It's interesting to me that I have had very few head colds or respiratory infections in the three or four years that I have been on this machine. I'm still trying to get skinny. Recently, I have heard of a small device, inserted into the nose that raises airway pressure slightly and improves sleep apnea. It will be great if this works out as CPAP machines are expensive and somewhat of a pain to use.

Chapter IX:

The Heart and Circulatory System

The heart was once known as the seat of the soul and of courage. Romantically and poetically, it still serves. "My heart is yours," or a name, as "Richard the Lionhearted", My Heart's in the Highlands."etc.

This organ's statistics are impressive in all species. For us, it beats 103,680 times in twenty-four hours, pumping approximately 7,200 liters of blood in a 180-mile circuit (in a 180-pound individual). It's capable of twice that rate for short periods in young, fit individuals. Rest? You really wouldn't want it to stop and rest. The only rest it gets is the pause between beats. It's muscle—highly specialized muscle—but it responds to exercise just as well as other muscle. It demands and gets the first oxygenated blood out of the lungs.

It has four chambers and four valves. The right atrium receives return blood from the body in the vena cava and primes the right ventricle to pump into the lungs. From there, blood enters the left atrium, which primes the left ventricle, which in turn powers the blood through the body via the arteries. Our systolic blood pressure is essentially the pressure within the left ventricle in its power stroke. When we were young and vigorous, our arteries were elastic and would expand with each heartbeat, smoothing out the pressure wave. Our diastolic blood pressure is the pressure between heartbeats. As we age, the vessels stiffen, become more rigid, and the pressure with each beat drops off quickly, producing the pounding we hear in our head at times. Blood pressure frequently rises with age, putting an increasing load on the heart. To some extent this is a compensating mechanism to allow increasing circulation to more distant and narrowing blood vessels. Concern about blood pressure is that the process gets out of control in a self-sustaining manner, putting an ever-increasing load on the heart and blood vessels, thereby causing damage. The damage, of course, is heart failure, heart attacks, strokes, and organ failure. Fortunately, over the last generation, we've had excellent medications that increase efficacy in blood pressure control (let's hear one good shout for the drug industry).

Heart Trouble

Coronary artery disease is one of our most frequent killers. Traditionally, it was mostly males who were afflicted with this, but the incidence has been steadily rising in females. It's thought that we are seeing the late results of more women smoking and of women in the stressful workplace. Smoking overall is decreasing in this country, and as a result we are seeing less cancer as well as less coronary artery disease, the root of which is the formation of calcium plaques and subsequent narrowing in the coronary arterial circulation. A lot of this is genetic. If you've had a parent or a close family member die in this manner, you need to be aware that you can't ignore this problem. Obesity is quickly becoming more of a causative factor as well, as is a sedentary lifestyle. You really can't get away from keeping your cholesterol low, blood pressure at a good level, and weight down, and avoiding tobacco and getting adequate exercise. Of course, the same thing applies to stroke avoidance.

Symptoms of a heart attack (acute coronary syndrome) include chest discomfort, which may be heavy and oppressive; pain in the left shoulder and arm; pain in the neck, jaw, and teeth; and shortness of breath. Some, all, or none of these may be present. Frequently, nausea is present, especially in women. Having observed the symptoms over the years and having dealt with some of them personally, I can urge without hesitation that these be investigated by your physician or in the emergency department. Sure, it can be something else, such as a backwash from the stomach or esophagitis, but why take a chance with something that can have a fatal outcome?

The aortic and mitral valves sometimes get deformed with age and disease. Occasionally, it can be genetic. A lot of this was caused by rheumatic fever in the past, which in turn was a progression of strep infections, usually in the tonsils. This is much less prevalent now that we have antibiotics, and more of these infections are treated early. These deformed valves leak, sometimes seriously, and can cause additional loads on the heart, resulting in heart failure. Replacement surgery is much better now. Heart failure is in itself a problem and is sometimes due to infection of the heart muscle. At times, multiple blockages of the small arteries can lead to heart failure as well.

Proceeding from the arterial side of circulation, blood flow goes through the capillary system. These are tiny, very fine blood vessels that can be so small as to allow one red blood cell at a time to march through. This is where oxygen-CO_2 exchange and other byproducts of metabolism take place. From there, the blood is collected into the system of veins, which, like river tributaries, join together in ever-increasing size to get back to the heart and lungs in the large vena cava. Most of the blood clots that we hear about originate in the veins. These are caused by stagnation of flow, injury, or inflammatory disease. Varicose veins are large and tortuous vessels frequently implicated in clots. We get more of these as we age. Small clots originating in the smaller vessels can travel up to the lungs where they're trapped and broken down, rarely causing consequences unless they come in showers. Larger clots, obviously, from larger veins are capable of causing serious impairment, even death.

Here's a pearl! When you are on a trip, stop the car every two hours, get out and walk around to flush out those veins! Helps drowsiness, too.

Arterial clots cut off the blood flow to the particular field that the occluded artery services, sometimes with disastrous consequences (e.g., major strokes, loss of function in kidneys, bowel, and limbs).

Obviously, anything we can do to prevent or slow the process of arteriosclerosis (hardening of our arteries) decreases the constant workload of the heart. Remember that overloading a machine makes the machine wear out faster. Intermittent workloads, like exercise, strengthen the organ. Weight loss seriously reduces the workload. The word is that each excess pound we carry requires a mile of blood vessels. Go figure.

Rest, particularly bed rest, weakens us. I'm not talking about that necessary eight hours here. While there's something to be said for rest and recuperation, I marvel at the old conventional wisdom, even in medical practice, of putting patients in bed to "gain strength". I can't help but wonder how much of our present-day health care is a matter of what is "currently fashionable." Ah, well... The older we are, the faster our bodies can lose strength at rest. Strength can't be saved. This weakening may be the worst result of an injury or illness affecting one part of our body and forcing rest on the total body, but resuming activity as soon as possible is the current good practice. So, here, again, is our old playmate exercise!

Chapter X:

The Liver, Gallbladder, and Pancreas

If the heart was the seat of the soul in ancient times, the liver was felt to be the seat of emotions. If you were of a sour disposition you were said to be "liverish" or "bilious." The liver was therefore assigned an important role, though for the wrong reason.

The liver is the body's primary chemical factory. It has an enormous blood supply for this purpose. It breaks down the products of digestion into basic usable compounds and manufactures an incredible number of substances we need in our body, such as cholesterol. That's right, we really do need it. Just the right kind and not so damn much of it. Sugars are changed into simple sugars or stored in the form of fat. The liver detoxifies various compounds that are dangerous for us, alcohol being one. It also detoxifies most of the medications that we use, through various enzyme systems. Along with the spleen, it takes tired beat-up blood cells out of circulation and recycles hemoglobin.

A major effort of the liver is the production of bile. This complex of organic salts is a necessity in the digestive tract. The liver produces this almost continuously. When it's not being squirted into the small intestine, it's diverted to storage in the gallbladder. Eating causes a contraction of this small, balloon-like organ under the liver and squirts additional bile into the gut just below the stomach. Bile is essential for breaking down fats.

Some of us have a tendency to form stones in the gall-bladder. In addition to causing pain, stones can actually block the bile duct. This brings about infection in the gall-bladder. If the stones go below that and block the common bile duct, bile backs up into the liver, causing liver cell destruction, pain, and infection, and that becomes an emergency, usually surgical. Uncomplicated gallbladder surgery is now done through a laparoscope with a small incision, and recovery is quick. Stones can sometimes be removed trough small tubes inserted into the gastrointestinal tract; complications can require the traditional incision. After the gallbladder is removed, bile flows continuously into the small bowel, causing diarrhea for a while. The longer surgery is put off, the worse complications can get.

There isn't too much that we need to dwell on about the spleen. It's about half the size of the palm of the hand and in the left side of the abdomen. Its two primary functions involve recycling red blood cells and enhancing the immune system. Its most common problem is injury due to trauma, rupture, and extensive hemorrhage, which can be life-threatening, due to its heavy-duty blood supply. Some leukemias can cause enlargement of the spleen, with increased danger of rupture. We can get along without the spleen, but need to pay extra attention to infection after its removal.

The pancreas is tucked deeply in the left side of the abdomen, and is a rather vital organ. It produces insulin, which we need to break down the sugars we eat, and it produces enzymes that are primarily involved with carbohydrate digestion. By far, the most common problem involving the pancreas is its failure to produce an adequate amount of insulin, which we need to break down sugars. This is diabetes. Diabetes is increasing—even in children—due to the overingestion of fats and sugars with concurrent obesity. Thanks to medical science and the ability of our drug industry, replacement of insulin and pancreatic enzymes is a long-standing, if moderate, success.

Perhaps the worst—certainly the sneakiest—pancreatic disease is cancer. Because of the remote location and modest chemical signatures, pancreatic cancer is usually rather advanced before it's detected. Treatment has been pretty much unsuccessful in the past, but seems to be improving. At least you don't suffer long with it. It's a good deal more frequent in male smokers and drinkers. Obesity may be a factor. Earlier diagnosis would be a big help.

Chapter XI:

The gut

The drive for food and nourishment is one of the primal urges of all life. Given this, it's understandable that so much attention has been paid to the digestive tract. I'm certain that there have been more volumes from a medical, as well as a lay, standpoint on the subject. While a lot of this is practical, down-to-earth stuff, a lot is just the fashion of the moment. Here's my attempt to cover the basics in a practical way. I've taken the liberty of including some of my opinions as well.

After food gets past the grinding mill of the teeth, the swallowing process begins, with the help of the tongue, and involves the esophagus. The esophagus is the muscular tube connecting the mouth and throat with the stomach. If you've ever watched a snake swallowing an egg or a mouse, you know exactly how the esophagus works. It squeezes above the food and relaxes below it in a continuous wave, pushing food and liquids down into the stomach.

If one is obese or has poor function of the valve at the top of the stomach, stomach acids can backwash into the esophagus, which has no protection of its own, and cause irritation, pain, and spasms. The pain can be severe enough to be confused with that of a heart attack. The spasm can cause the temporary blockage of food, which in itself can be quite uncomfortable. After years of abuse with stomach acids and corrosives such as alcohol, the esophagus gradually loses its function. Heartburn occurs when stomach acid and digestive juices backwash into the esophagus and burn the esophageal lining, which has no layer of mucus protecting it as does the stomach. Sometimes the valve at the top of the stomach is incompetent due to a hiatal hernia (a portion of the stomach extending up through the diaphragm), and sometimes the backwash occurs because of a full stomach and position of the body such as lying down. Obviously, anything that causes an increase in stomach acid production and churning, such as unresolved stress, aggravates the whole situation. The esophagus can go into spasm, locking up the swallowing process. This is uncomfortable and can cause severe pain in the chest. Again, it is one of the "rule outs" when thinking of angina and coronary artery disease.

Sensible eating, not reclining too soon after eating, and elevating the head of the bed on four- to six-inch blocks can be helpful. Antacids are also helpful, but the acid blockers have proven to be the most effective. Remember, though, that your primary medical caregiver should evaluate any condition that is undiagnosed or persists for a while.

Cancer of the esophagus (a mean beast) occurs much more frequently in men who smoke and have a heavy alcohol intake. Let's talk about the process of swallowing a little bit more. Most of the time, this is an automatic process. Food and liquid that we ingest is passed into the esophagus. Usually, the flap valve (epiglottis) blocking the airway works so that we don't inhale food or liquid into the airway. We're hearing a lot more about heartburn now that the acid blockers have gone generic and over the counter. They do work well. Again, a tip of the hat to the pharmaceutical industry

The stomach is one of the more remarkable organs in the body. I've always had a great deal of respect for the manner in which it takes a lot of abuse and continues to work. Structurally, it's a sack with valves at each end. The stomach lining secretes acid and digestive enzymes such as pepsin (which breaks down protein), and a thick mucus that protects the stomach from digesting itself. After a meal, a churning action takes place to help mix and digest the food. Anxiety and tobacco increase churning and acid production. Some substances, such as alcohol, thin the mucus coating. This allows the stomach to self-digest in areas, producing—guess what? Ulcers! Fortunately, the pharmaceutical industry is again able to come to our rescue with effective medications.

Leaving the stomach through the pyloric valve, the food stream, now liquefied, passes into the duodenum, gets a squirt of bile from the gallbladder, enters the jejunum, and then moves into the ileum. The churning and mixing continue, and most of the absorption of the products of digestion takes place here. The small bowel is free of a lot of pathology excepting the duodenum, just below the stomach, which can ulcerate. Inflammatory bowel disease is not extremely common, but can be a booger. Gluten intolerance—a sensitivity to wheat products affecting the small bowel that can be present from birth—seems to be becoming more frequent, but perhaps it's being diagnosed more often.

Another valve, and the digestive liquids pass into the colon. A primary action here is the recycling of water. This is absorbed from the now-fecal stream and put back in service to assist the body's fluid balance. The colon is a good bit larger in diameter than the small bowel and lies along the right side of the abdomen, swags over the top to the left side of the abdomen, descends, and then, after a few twists and turns of the sigmoid area, goes into the rectum. The colon has the same "snake swallowing" action as the rest of the gut, having similar muscle fibers in its wall. For some reason, unknown to me, it has small fatty tags on its outer wall. In many of us, the inner lining herniates into these tags, producing little pockets called diverticula. These sometimes will block off and become infected (diverticulitis), a chronic inflammatory process with pain and fever, similar to that of appendicitis, but on the left side. They can bleed as well, sometimes acutely. Also, a fair number of us have the genetic code that produces internal growths, called polyps, in the colon. Left alone, these can develop into colon cancer. This is the primary reason we're cautioned to get a colonoscopy exam,periodically, after age 50. It's nice to know that colon cancer is decreasing in our population because of this.

Cancers do develop in the sigmoid area and rectum. Most of these are well within reach of the rectal examiner's finger. Hey, we don't like to do that exam any more than you like to have it done. Good cleansing of the rectal area is important and can help an individual detect a developing growth. The more frequent problem is the development of varicose veins around the rectum, which can clot off and cause very aggravating pain and discomfort. These are caused by constipation or sitting on the commode, straining, for long periods. There really are more comfortable places to read a magazine. The straining and pressure with childbirth causes this in women. We're talking hemorrhoids here. Rectal itching and burning is not due to hemorrhoids, but inflammation. Pain during defecation usually indicates a split in the skin of the rectum itself, which can happen with constipation.

The rectum itself really is a remarkable, if somewhat unappreciated, organ. It's suspended by a funnel-shaped organization of muscle and surrounded by circular muscle bands. These, with the help of a very complex system of innervation, give a refined degree of control for all of us. This control tends to decrease as we age, so be careful! It can separate gas, liquids, and solids to an amazing degree, unlike some birds, that poop with a gravitational stimulus. Watch out for seagulls when they pull up after diving!

Over the years, volumes have been written about bowel function. Some of us get to the point of obsession with bowel activity and feel that they are ill if the daily bowel movement does not fill a bushel basket. Well, that is an overstatement, but it was a subject that I encountered frequently in my family practice. Many of the perceived problems that we have from digestion to defecation begin in childhood. I remember one bright three-year-old girl pointing to her stool, which was circling the commode and about to disappear, angrily saying, "Mine, mine." She was upset over a loss of a body part, not recognizing it as waste at her age.

I've often wondered how much of our chronic constipation is due to being forced to sit on the potty until something happens. Young children are frequently just too busy to take the time for a bowel movement. They will wait until they involuntarily fill their pants, or worse, wait until the fecal material dries out and becomes hard, large, and painful to pass. Of course, this becomes a painful cycle. In times past, your parents may have been almost frantic at making sure their children had a daily bowel movement. These people have used childhood laxatives to an excessive degree. These concerns become personalized and can carry on to adulthood. It really isn't necessary to have a daily bowel movement to be healthy, nor is it necessary to have a large, copious stool. Much of the trouble comes from chronic laxative use, again, some of which dates back to childhood. The more frequently laxatives are used, the more dependent the bowel will become on them. In extreme cases, a dependence on enemas develops. I don't wish to say that occasional laxatives, even enemas, are not needed. Stool softeners are preferable, and an adequate fluid intake is necessary.

A couple of centuries ago, physicians were acutely aware of the character and quality of the bowel movement. Indeed, even at present many pathologic conditions can be diagnosed in this manner. The era of the microscope and bacteriology ushered in even more intense examination. Routine testing is done for the presence of blood at the time of your physical. Cultures done during an illness can detect the presence of disease organisms. I think most people are unaware that we have an incredibly large universe of microorganisms in the gut. These help with digestion and absorption of vitamins and other necessary substances and comprise a fair amount of bulk in the stool.

Our diet and fluid intake have more to do with bowel activity than anything else. We're hearing a lot in recent years about high-fiber diets. This is good stuff. Fiber in the diet decreases diverticular disease and cancer of the bowel. These two problems are virtually unknown in primitive societies that ingest a lot of vegetable fiber and fruit in their diet. I remember reading that some African tribes have a large number of bowel movements on this kind of an intake. It's interesting, though, that fiber seems to regulate the overactive bowel as well. I haven't seen much research on this, but I do know that some individuals who have frequent loose bowel movements, even some degree of griping and fecal incontinence are able to slow bowel activity down to the point of having formed, controllable stools with a daily dose of an over-the-counter fiber product. The amount of liquid intake with the fiber may need to be decreased.

As we age, the digestive tract loses some of its ability to break down carbohydrates. These carbohydrates tend to ferment and they produce—guess what—gas! A fair amount of this is methane. Here we are at the very literal essence of being an "old fart." Some foods such as beans—the musical fruit—are worse than others in producing gas. And we do swallow a fair amount of the gas that we expel. Most of this we burp out, but some passes through. We can observe this aerophagia easily with various imaging techniques. It's particularly noticeable with swallowing fluids.

Chapter XII:

The Urinary Tract

We continue the discussion about excretion, this time of fluids. For starters, think of the kidneys as filters. We have two kidneys, one on each side, deep in the upper abdomen. Instead of filtering out solids, they remove the waste product—urea—some proteins, and some toxins as well. They adjust levels of calcium salts and other soluble compounds while maintaining proper fluid balance in our bodies. All of our blood is in continuous flow through the kidneys. Incidentally, if that blood flow is mechanically restricted (atherosclerotic plaques or birth anomalies), one gets a mean case of high blood pressure. This is not the usual cause of hypertension, however.

If the concentration of the filtered substances gets too high in that part of the kidney devoted to collection, crystals can form. Remember basic chemistry? Well, the saturated solutions form crystals, which grow larger and become kidney stones. Urologists tell us that keeping the urine dilute (i.e., near colorless) is a major help in avoiding stones. Drink your eight glasses of water daily. The urine trickles down from the kidneys through little tubes called ureters into the bladder, a major source of woe as we age. The prostate gland, usually about the size of a walnut, encircles the urethra, which is a tube leading from the bladder through the penis. This (that is, the gland, not the penis) frequently enlarges as the male ages and causes narrowing and back pressure in the urinary tract. The bladder stretches, and doesn't empty as well as it did. Muscle fibers change into scar tissue, which has no ability to contract and empty the bladder. Infections of the urethra, such as gonorrhea, can cause scarring and narrowing of this tubular structure, as well as affecting other areas of the reproductive system. This can usually be dealt with if detected early.

I've laid out the structure and normal function of the urinary tract. This tract is the source of a lot of the frustration us males have with getting older. Not that our female counterparts don't have their share of problems with this system, but after all, this is a sexist document.

We really don't appreciate being able to pee across the creek when we are kids. I suppose this is where the phrase "pissing contest" originated. When the bladder is small with good, young, muscle, it can contract to an amazing degree, producing a strong flow. Conversely, as we age, the bladder stretches, and the muscle fibers weaken and become partially replaced with scar tissue and then the bladder doesn't empty as well.

The fact that the bladder empties at all is good. Remember the prostate gland that encircles the urethra, that tube that leads from the bladder through the penis? When this gland enlarges, as it frequently does with age, it restricts and can even completely shut off urinary flow from the bladder. This makes for bad times, with a lot of pain and discomfort and a strong urge to urinate. The back pressure on the urinary tract causes damage to all parts above, particularly the kidneys. A complete blockage, or even high-grade partial blockage, has to be relieved. Nowadays, this is temporarily done with a flexible catheter (a tube that is pushed into the bladder through the urethra). I remember chronically enlarged bladders holding two liters or more of urine. That hurts to even think about it. Fortunately, there are several procedures that can be done to take care of this kind of obstruction, including complete or partial removal of the prostate gland, surgery, freezing, and lasers. The difficult part is maintaining some level of control over urination, not to mention preserving sexual activity, after these procedures. Believe me, though, if you have urinary obstruction, you'll want it relieved, whatever the consequences.

The opposite of urinary retention is urinary incontinence. While this does occur as overflow incontinence (the bladder is full and can't hold any more), it most often happens because of a loss of control of the valve (sphincter) at the base of the bladder. The more minor, but nonetheless aggravating, problem that we face with an aging urinary tract is that of dribbling, incomplete emptying, and partial incontinence. Even for young males, it's difficult to end urination with complete dryness. That's impossible as we age. Another area of frustration is that of a weak urinary stream. It becomes difficult to predict where this weak stream will go. Some of this is due to the fact that the urethra shrinks in length, becomes more tortuous, or both. Couple this with weak outflow pressure, and the urinary stream can even flow back up over the genital area. Nothing is safe anywhere within a 180-degree half circle in front of you and a few degrees back between your feet. The urine frequently ends up on the floor or on your clothing. This, of course, leads to the many pithy words of advice found scribbled above the commode in public places, such as, "It's shorter than you think; step up closer, please." By the way, if you really want to make your significant other mad, don't lift the seat before you urinate.

I remember some years ago that Japanese homes had a small urinal mounted at an appropriate height on the wall of their restrooms. That seemed very sensible, and I've often wondered why we didn't have some similar appliance in our country. Do realize that you're not alone. All males will have some problem with urination if they're fortunate enough to live that long. It really shouldn't be a cause of embarrassment. There are absorbent undergarments, and washing machines are plentiful. Hey, we can always sit. It's terribly important, as was pointed out in the section on appearance and self-respect, to be clean, dry, and free of odor. As it turns out, older women are more troubled with episodic incontinence than are men.

When the bladder doesn't empty completely, the possibility of a urinary tract infection rises. As in the case with all body cavities, good drainage is essential. This is why collections of infection in the body known as abscesses have been healed when they finally erupt to the outside and drain. Over the ages, medicine men learned that the technique of opening and draining was curative. Hence, the old expression "laudable pus." Nowadays, the surgeon or ER doc will place a temporary drain in an area that is likely to become infected.

One really doesn't want to have a bladder or other urinary tract infection, as they can be very destructive. Chronic urinary tract infections can actually destroy kidney function over the years and some bad acute infections can do the kidneys in, as well as cause a serious systemic infection that can be fatal.

One of the best things we can do for urinary health is to drink plenty of water. Eight glasses per day is said to be about right. If you drink enough to keep the urine stream near colorless, you're about right. If you have to strain to urinate, you have waited too long in visiting the urologist. Obstruction occurs gradually and there are several procedures available before extensive surgery is required. Blood in the urine requires evaluation. Sudden pain in either flank or in the pubic area (a calling card of the kidney stone) will get your attention, also.

It continues to be said that a lot of men will die with cancer of the prostate. Please notice that I said with and not of. This simply means that almost all men will develop cancer of the prostate if they live long enough. Occasionally, men do die of advanced cancer of the prostate. It can be an aggressive disease in the younger male, under sixty or thereabouts. After age seventy, it's usually rather slow growing. There's considerable debate as to whether or not it should be treated if it is slow growing. The options range from complete surgical removal to shrinkage with cryosurgery (freezing) or radiation. Anti hormonal (antitestosterone) therapy has been a hallmark of treatment over the years. Needless to say, it's always important to get appropriate specialty opinions.

In any event, one really doesn't want to become that old fart that smells of stale urine and dirty clothing. Keep the washing machine busy if that's what it takes.

Chapter XIII:

Sexual Activity and the Old Fart

Hah! I'll bet that most of you turned to this chapter first. Well, we've been talking about the urinary tract, which is somewhat important in sexual function. Actually, it might've been more appropriate if this discussion followed this section on the activity of the brain; the brain is the biggest sexual organ that we have.

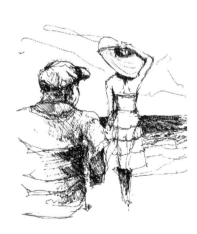

Not only do we think about sex—hells bells, we're preoccupied with it, all of us. In spite of what we hear from the media about our society's incessant focus on sex, we're not the first. Reproduction is the most basic instinct of any species. For us humans, this is revealed by classic ancient writers thousands of years before Christ. When these literati weren't writing poetic odes about lopping off each other's heads and limbs, wading knee-deep in gore and guts, and chucking massy spears at each other, they homed in on the sexual exploits of their heroes, particularly the gods. Rape seemed to be preferable to usual sexual activity; they didn't seem to have time for foreplay, but I suppose the spectacular was preferred then as now. The gods were particularly active in the rape of various nymphs and naiads, as well as humankind. *The Days of Our Gods* would've been the prime title of the ancient soap opera, if indeed they had soap. And even before the written word, all of the above was passed down orally by those aged bards who were much revered themselves. Then, too, it's been a much noted casus belli, as per the Trojan War, and the rape of the Sabine women.

Never think that interest in the opposite sex gradually disappears as we climb through our advancing years. One of the worst flirts I ever met was a bedridden, ninety-two-year-old widow. She delighted in my house calls (yes, I did make them), saying, "Oh, here comes my good-looking doctor," and patting the side of the bed for me to sit on. I didn't look too shabby back in those days. We would have a wonderful visit. I've personally observed my wonderful ninety-year-old mother-in-law admiring a buff young male, particularly if he had a cute butt. And I really don't know many older males, myself included, who fail to appreciate a lovely, well-turned-out lass in a bikini, or one just nicely dressed, for that matter. When I fail to notice some female's lovely legs, narrow waist, and well-contoured breasts, just throw a few handfuls of earth over me because I'm already gone.

Sexual activity does indeed change—make that decrease—as we age. I've heard the wry comment that it'd be a lot better if your sexual equipment fell off instead of your teeth falling out. I think it's Falstaff who opines in one of Shakespeare's King Henry plays that age does geld a man. One of the more common things that happen to many of us is a decrease in the amount of testosterone produced by the testes. We're beginning to see references to this by the pharmaceutical industry promoting their snake oil. And, indeed, there are various forms of replacement available. Perhaps even more important than the decrease in libido, things like energy level, stamina, and depression are caused in part by the lower levels of this hormone. The anabolic (bodybuilding) hormones that are illegally used in sports are related to testosterone. It's interesting that the administration of testosterone and these other hormones can cause the testes to shrink, although the penis can maintain size and erectile ability. I don't know about you, but I'm a lot more interested in function than in cosmetics.

The penis is a remarkable organ in the healthy state, and with good blood supply. It has the ability to engorge and erect to several times its resting state. Young males, who are sometimes said to think with their testicles, maintain a resting state in the penis larger than do elderly males. Maybe that's for purposes of quick draw. As we age, erections are less frequent and less turgid. More and longer stimulation is required. There's no organ in the male body more susceptible to psychological state of mind as is the penis. If the least doubt of your ability to achieve or maintain an erection flashes through the brain, forget it—you're done. This happens even in younger males, and is the cause of a great deal of angst, as well as the most frequent cause of impotence. Incidentally, if you awaken with the nocturnal erection, the mechanical equipment is okay. If you don't know whether or not this happens, there's an old, simple test that you can use privately. Simply take a strip of postage stamps (you don't need expensive ones) and stick them around the flaccid penis at bedtime. If the strip is broken in the morning—voilà!—you have your answer.

If you take the time to read the litany of side effects that accompany your prescription medications, you'll find that almost every one of them mentions an interference with sexual activity. They're talking about the ability to achieve and maintain an erection, of course. This doesn't mean that your medication shouldn't be taken. After all, some degree of control of strokes, heart attacks, and high blood pressure is of more importance to health and longevity than penile penetration, the frequency of which declines as we age anyway. Certainly, this is worth a discussion with your physician. There may be an alternative medication. And keep in mind that there are many ways of giving and receiving sexual satisfaction. Use your imagination.

As noted in the above, erectile dysfunction (or "ED," as snake oil salesmen love to call it) is now widely trumpeted in the advertising media and by various persons of note. I suspect that there are very few males who don't have at least occasional difficulty with this at some time during their lives. An important thing that I can leave you with is that you shouldn't regard this as a cataclysmic event that means the end of your sex life. Again, think of that largest and most important sexual organ that you possess, the brain. If it perceives adequate sexual arousal, it will carry you a long way.

I'm absolutely serious about this. Arousal is triggered easily in younger males but is more deeply buried as we get older. As noted above, it takes longer to achieve a state of arousal. But, on the other hand, it may be more satisfying. It certainly is more appreciated, being more

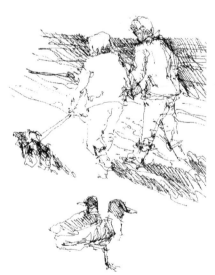

infrequent. One other thing, orgasm doesn't need to happen every time. There's a lot of sexual satisfaction in cuddling and caressing. By the way, achieving orgasm takes longer as we get older, too. Assuming that a certain level of physical fitness is present, this can be a good thing.

Speaking of the medications for ED, I once asked a preteen nephew what he thought about these television advertisements. He said,

"It means you just get your confidence up and go for it!" I don't think he knew exactly what he was saying, but it was a pretty good description. These drugs are a big income producer for the pharmaceutical industry. This isn't unusual. Aphrodisiacs have been a major item of commerce from day one. There are some animal species, notably bears, tigers, and the rhinoceros, that are being pushed to extinction by the demand from impotent, elderly Asian males seeking these animals' gallbladder and powdered horns, respectively. If any of these aphrodisiacs worked well, there wouldn't be so damn many of them. The newer drugs work by increasing the amount of a chemical that's necessary for penile engorgement. They certainly can be helpful if one can get around the side effects, which can be very annoying and counterproductive. They'll all tell you to seek medical attention if an erection lasts longer than four hours. Wow, don't you wish! Actually, that would be rather painful. Another thing, maybe I'm stupid, but I still haven't figured out the significance of lying around in two old bathtubs.

Many—perhaps most—of us find that being in a warm emotional relationship with our significant other is the most necessary part of sexual activity and satisfaction. Long gone are the days when "Roll over," was foreplay. Women have always been more sensitive in this regard than men. Just like the male, the menopausal and postmenopausal female undergoes a decrease in hormonal activity resulting in decreased libido. Incidentally, males may not go through menopause per se, but many of us experience a male climacteric. (Sounds better, doesn't it). Seems to me it amounts to much the same. The environment and emotional temperature of the relationship are very important. If there is anger, too much stress, or a lot of anxiety in the situation, sexual coupling may take place, but it probably won't be very satisfying. This can go all the way to "Are you done yet?"

What this means is that one needs to be a motivated, caring lover. Bringing a bouquet of flowers home once a month ain't gonna do it! Cooking a meal, washing dishes, or at least helping out in the cleanup, and doing a load of laundry on occasion all work pretty well. So does a movie and a romantic dinner at a nice restaurant. Be spontaneous; use your imagination. Your partner needs to know that you really do care, that you really do consider him or her desirable, and that you're sensitive to wants and needs, and not just in an episodic manner, either. Sure, this road has two ends that meet, but it doesn't hurt to do whatever is necessary.

You've noticed, I'm sure, that I'm not trying to write a sex manual here. There are lots of those around already, dating back to antiquity and existing in other cultures. The sexual relationship between two people is and should be very private, and hopefully satisfying. And despite many authoritative efforts to proscribe certain sexual behaviors over the ages, it's always been a truism that what works between two individuals is their business. But, I repeat, it must be good for both. And it stands to reason that "kiss and tell," or any variation thereof, is an absolute no-no.

Well, it's long been said that love is wasted on the young. The same applies to sexual activity. But it's also true that there are a lot of things we don't appreciate well until we're older and perhaps have more time for contemplation. One can find a world of pithy quotations to the effect that a bad marriage is one of the most beastly things that can happen to two people. There are equal numbers stating that a good marriage is the most sublime of relationships. Compatibility and companionship are incredibly important, as is the ability to communicate with each other. Many of us do indeed find our soul mates, and that's wonderful, indeed. Just because a couple achieves that level in a relationship doesn't mean that they can relax and stay that way forever. It takes ongoing care, concern, and work to maintain. Worth it? .....Damn right!

Chapter XIV

That Wonderful Organ the Skin

No organism on Earth could exist without some form of covering and containment; ours is our skin. In addition to being our chief protection from the environment, it's a major factor in the control of our body temperature. It's an excretory organ as well, elaborating sweat and oils. The process of sweating is part of temperature control.

The skin is extremely flexible, allowing us our tremendous range of motion. Its ability to darken or tan gives us protection from those rays of the sun that are harmful. Witness those races that live in equatorial regions. Over the eons, they've developed darker skin, without which they wouldn't have survived as well. Conversely, those of us who've lived in temperate or more northern (or extreme southern) zones tend to get along with a complexion that is lighter. Of course, the lighter you are, the more sensitive you are to sunburn, which is the initial skin response to damaging radiant energy. Part of the skin's flexibility is due to the fats and oils that it produces. Genetic changes that lack this ability produce a skin that cracks and fissures, sometimes extensively.

The skin has the ability to heal cuts and damage rather quickly with scar tissue. It's constantly renewing itself with the outer cells of the epidermis flaking off and new cells pushing up. Surgical repair of lacerations has been done since very ancient times, more in some societies than others. Several means of closure have been used, even using the pinching heads of large ants. Linen and silk sutures have also been used, as were the boiled hairs of horse mane and tail. While they were boiled to make them flexible, that had the unrealized advantage of making them sterile. Medical people in ancient cultures of India even practiced cosmetic surgery on the face.

Obviously, large lacerations to the limbs and body healed with better function and less scarring when the tissues were approximated. Roman military surgeons were quite good at this, reaching a degree of excellence not achieved again until the late eighteenth century. Nothing's new, is it? Hopefully, we keep rediscovering history and making use of it.

The skin, of course, produces hair. There are specialized skin cells that do this. I suspect most body hair is vestigial and is gradually disappearing from Homo sapiens. I don't know this, but I suspect that pubic hair has a sexual function. Hair on the scalp has an obvious protective function. Hair in the ears and nasal passages help keep critters out. Eyelashes protect the eyes, and it seems reasonable that eyebrows have a function in communication. For that matter, the skin itself communicates—think of blushing and goose pimples.

Skin Conditions

I've mentioned elsewhere the importance of the various skin cancers. The basal-cell cancer usually presents as a nonhealing ulcer that isn't painful. It doesn't metastasize to other areas of the body; it just grows and can become disfiguring. The squamous-cell carcinoma can be mean, metastasize, and cause systemic disease. These are more often flat, scaly, nonhealing areas, usually dark in color and irregular in shape. Melanomas are the sneaky ones.

They're brownish red to dark, even black, in color. Most of us have many freckles of various shades. You should be concerned if they change shape or color, but if there's any question, a physician should be consulted. They're easily excised when found early, and an adequate border taken around them. One other, more unusual presentation is under the nails, where they can appear as a dark spot or line that persists.

Many of us develop soft fleshy growths on the skin. If these papillomas are left alone, they can enlarge. They're not very pretty, but they're not dangerous. One older woman, opining on the internet said that some of her skin growths had gotten so large, she had named them. Of course, we have warts, usually in our younger years. As we get older, we develop the raised flaky patches of solar keratosis. They may itch. They're usually smaller than the similar patches of psoriasis, and are a cosmetic problem. Psoriasis is an interesting skin problem that seems to get worse with unresolved stress and better with sun exposure. Fungi are opportunists and come and go. Persistent fungal infections can herald diabetes. Dermatologists can be very helpful with all of the above.

Bathing

Over the ages there has been incredible economic activity related to cosmetics, bathing, and protection from the sun, which, of course, includes clothing. It's interesting that the ancient Romans and Greeks didn't have soap, but used hot and cold baths, scraping the skin, and applying oils, at least in the upper classes. Up until relatively recent times, bathing wasn't considered to be necessary for hygiene. I would guess that perfumes and lotions were much in demand in those days. A word about bathing: As skin gets older, its ability to furnish lubrication decreases remarkably. If we bathe daily with our efficient detergent soaps, particularly in the dry wintertime, our skin can get dry and itchy. Most of us use a daily shower and shampoo. For some it's better to soap and scrub in the underarm, genital, facial, arm, and hand areas daily, then every few days do a total body scrub followed by a bath. As an alternative, you might get by using a lotion containing soap; some of these are liquid. A dandruff shampoo containing conditioner is helpful as well. Be careful with bath oils and lotions in the tub and shower—they're slick, and these are frequent places for falls.

Chapter XV:

Pills, Potions, and Poisons

Our society is the most heavily medicated in history. This fact isn't even arguable, to buzz an overused word. It seems to be characteristic of Homo sapiens that we've searched for magic elixirs, cures for real and supposed illnesses, pain relievers, and tranquilizers since the beginning of our time on this planet. Any magic elixirs have eluded me, but an incredible store of folk knowledge has built up over many thousands of years about various plants and minerals that have medicinal properties. Unfortunately, much, perhaps even most, of this knowledge has been lost. We've always had shamans, witch doctors, "yarb" (herb) doctors, and grannies that've passed their knowledge down through generations. Independent researchers, as well as those employed by the pharmaceutical industry, are frantically seeking to recapture this knowledge and to discover new compounds that might be of use in our society or be an economic commodity.

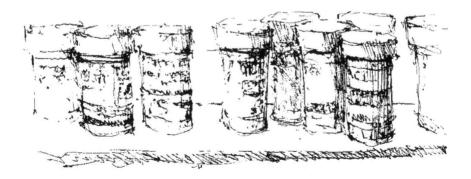

And, yes, the snake oil salesmen are still with us. We read about these people in our histories and used to see them touting nostrums from the backs of their wagons in our western movies. Nowadays, they're after us on television, in our magazines, and on billboards. They're shameless. Thank goodness for the little bit of regulation that we do have. One has to remember that their primary purpose is to coax you into buying their products. I especially deplore the advertising of prescription medications. Of course, they all say you must consult—make that harass—your doctor about writing these prescriptions. And to conform to the Federal Drug Administration's rules, all of them chant a litany of side effects that are almost all the same. By the way, if you really listen to these side effects, you would hesitate to take any of these medications. Or they might specify that the medication should only be taken before bedtime on the first Tuesday past the full moon. Another favorite snake oil tactic is to convince you that you're the victim of some disease that can only be helped by their product. I'm talking about everything from cosmetics and soaps to prescription medication.

Forgive me if I long for the days before advertising of prescription drugs was a feature of our society. Within my lifetime, most of the pharmaceutical companies were owned and controlled by families who seemed to have rather strict ethical standards. Certainly, they promoted their products, but only to physicians. They advertised in medical journals and sponsored scientific seminars. One had the feeling that these companies were more interested in producing bona fide medications for the good of mankind than in reaping every last of the almighty dollar. Of course, doctors, and for that matter, lawyers didn't advertise in those days either. Oh well!

I have to say that academic and pharmaceutical researchers have done a marvelous job. I suspect that at least 75 percent of the medications now in use, which are, for the most part, very effective, weren't available when I began practice in the 1960s. The profit motive isn't all bad, unless too keenly applied. The pharmaceutical companies scream that their high prices are necessary for their very expensive research and development of new drugs. This is a fallacious argument. Any industry has to invest in research and development to survive, and the drug industry is no different. Another argument that's used is that high drug prices are necessary to support those medications that have a limited market due to the relative rarity of the targeted diseases. One only has to look at the incredible prices charged for these medications—sometimes many thousands of dollars per year—to realize that this, too, is a hollow claim. When one examines drug prices in other countries, particularly in those that have an organized health care system, it's readily apparent that their overall cost for drugs is lower. I suspect that we wouldn't mind supporting lower cost for medications in developing countries, particularly those medications used for AIDS and other epidemics. Organized health systems are able to negotiate lower prices, and I, for one, see no reason that this country shouldn't be in there negotiating as well.

The time involved and the cost of developing new drugs are quite substantial. Some of this is due to bureaucratic regulations. Many of these regulations are necessary to do the pretty good job of protecting our public from shoddy drugs, wildly exaggerated claims of efficacy, and counterfeit manufacturing. The pharmaceutical companies complain loudly about the limitations of the drug patent process, but they protect their patents like an eagle protects their young. They do all sorts of reformulations and minor changes to their drugs to extend the patent. Once the patent runs out, the generic manufacturers are let loose. They're supposed to be inspected and regulated as closely as the patent-protected manufacturers. Some of the major pharmaceutical companies have a cozy relationship with and even own generic plants, and, of course, can continue manufacture of the same drug, in a generic or over-the-counter form. It's worth noting that the retail pharmacies love generic drugs because the profit margin is greater. Of course, we, the consumer, are delighted to get our medications at a lower price. I've been on the same medicines for so long that all but one of them is generic. I have to say that many times these expensive medications help to avoid even more expensive hospitalizations. But...whatever the market will bear, right?

I want to check on this, but I believe that the market for consumer products that have to do with health and appearance is in excess of that for prescription drugs. This, of course, extends to food supplements, vitamins, and pain relievers. This is where the die-hard snake oil salesmen thrive. An incredible portion of the advertising industry is involved in promoting these products. There's no question that many of these products work well. Personally, I would hate to do without some of the over-the-counter pain relievers or antacids or bowel stimulants (not laxatives) that we're exposed to. Possibly, the best we can do is to take some of these exaggerated claims of efficacy with a grain of salt, realize that there's a placebo effect in everything, and do the best we can. Many times, an ice pack or a hot pack will work just fine. I remember being told in medical school years ago that most illnesses would resolve themselves If you could avoid harming the patient. Sometimes this calls for judgment, and that's where training as a medical professional comes in.

In ancient times, one could purchase charms, philters, potions, and poisons to accomplish almost anything. You could cast a spell of destruction, make the object of your affection fall hopelessly in love with you, cure various illnesses, and, of course, kill people. Excepting poisons, none of these worked too well, except in the mind of the user. It's wild that these things—again excepting out-and-out poisons—are still with us and vigorously promoted in tabloid publications, TV, and junk e-mails. Let's face it, if any of the promotions for penile enlargement worked, it would found a business that would dwarf the computer industry. Pretty much the same can be said of the other promotions. I believe that the only thing that works for male baldness, to a degree, started out as a prescription drug. These products are advertised for one reason—to take money away from you.

Smoking

Let's talk a little bit about the poisons to which we're commonly exposed in our society and environment. There's only one of these whose use is diminishing in the United States. That's tobacco. It's a marvelously addictive substance for most of us. It's a common foundation for lung disease in smokers and cancer of the mouth and stomach in all users, and is a causative factor in multiple other cancers, including breast and bowel. A person's life span is said to be shortened by anywhere from five to fifteen years. This doesn't seem like much when we are in our twenties and thirties, but when we approach the end of life; we realize that it's one hell of a lot. I've mentioned this before, but people have the idea that the ax will fall, that sudden death five to fifteen years early might not be all that bad. For the huge majority of us, it doesn't happen that way. We spend those last years smothering to death and in chronic pain or discomfort, not to mention disability. And, of course, the health care costs are considerable.

Alcohol

Alcohol is another booger. This has been around since day one. Fermentation is one of the basic chemical processes. It's a marvel to me that we've been able to evolve to the degree that we have in spite of ethyl alcohol. For almost all of history, alcohol has been used as medicine.

It's been used in religious ceremonies. Its use to excess has generally been denounced in all societies, most particularly in those more civilized. Beer and wine were common beverages in ancient times and safer to drink than water. The Romans used a heavy red wine, acetum, as an effective, antibacterial, wound irrigation. Distillation gave us alcohol in a more concentrated form, more toxic and faster acting but otherwise the same as the fermented beverages. Concentrated alcohols are flammable, used as fuels, and some are extremely toxic, such as methyl alcohol, taking out the brain and liver rather quickly. They're a painful bactericidal substance, but they also damage tissue in high concentrations.

Alcohol certainly was among our earliest tranquilizers, but ancient herbalists used others. It actually has an excitatory effect as well. For example, an average-size person can detoxify one ounce of ethyl alcohol per hour. As long as alcohol is in the system, it depresses (tranquilizes) the nervous system. After this, there is a ten- to twelve-hour spell of hyperactivity that can be uncomfortable and require additional sedation. This is why we wake up in the middle of the night after a few drinks and why we feel our nerves jangled in a hangover. This is believed to be one of the mechanisms that lead to addiction. It's also true that in some individuals, depression of the nervous systems leads immediately to wildly erratic, and even psychotic, behavior (Dr. Jekyll and Mr. Hyde?). This seems to be truer of distilled alcohol than of the fermented variety, but it certainly can happen either way. Judgment is impaired. One drink leads to another, or as Alcoholics Anonymous says, "One is too many and one hundred isn't enough." The tendency toward alcohol addiction runs in families. It's said that one alcoholic parent will produce the tendency for addiction in 50 percent of the children. I don't even want to think about what happens with two alcoholic parents. It would seem that prohibition of alcohol would be reasonable. It's been tried, of course, and it was a social disaster. We do like to relax with that beer, glass of wine, or cocktail in the evening, but, we have to always keep in mind that alcohol is one of the prime factors in dysfunctional and broken families and in spousal and child abuse. The fact that this can happen in an alcoholic blackout doesn't forgive the action. Legally, we do make the conscious choice to imbibe.

I've seen several articles to the effect that we elders can slip very easily into excessive alcohol use. We may be retired and not have schedules to keep or have as many responsibilities. We love to relax and have a friendly drink with friends. The aches and pains of arthritis are somewhat relieved with alcohol. There are usually more social activities available to us, many involving the use of alcohol. Alcohol does exert a toxic effect on the brain. Research studies have shown that alcohol ingestion causes the death of brain cells, perhaps even with modest drinking. We know that we also lose brain tissue and function as we age. It's sadly true that we don't detoxify alcohol as well as we age. This can be a scenario for disaster. We're in the process of losing coordination and balance as well as muscular strength, anyway. We dread falls and subsequent injuries. Our ability to react quickly to an emergency, such as those happening while driving, decreases with age. Certainly, this is a very variable thing. It happens to some of us early in life. There are those who aren't affected much at an advanced age. Old farts have to be cautious and careful, and exercise considerable restraint. Enough said.Then again, moderate use of alcohol seems to confer some health benefits. But how did you keep those who have a tendency for addiction at a moderate level? Alcohol education and the earliest possible treatment are partial answers. Total, lifelong abstinence seems to be the only real solution for those at risk. It's long been known that a high percentage of our prison population is due to crimes committed under the influence of alcohol and other addictions. And, again, think of health care costs, not to mention the sickening amount of death and injury due to operating a motor vehicle under the influence of alcohol.

Drugs

Well, what about the other poisons? No less familiar than alcohol, the illegal drugs, amphetamines, cocaine, and opiates, along with pot and hash are constantly in the news. There are continuing efforts to legalize marijuana for medical purposes. In places where this is successful, the process seems to me to be abused. Marijuana does seem to have a soporific and pain relieving effect on cancer and other chronic illness. Perhaps the future there will be some way that the specific chemicals involved can be incorporated into prescription medications. I was fairly adventurous as a kid, getting into alcohol at an early age. Had marijuana been available, I probably would have tried it. I certainly couldn't wait to smoke tobacco. It was pounded into us, though, that using marijuana was a quick downhill slide into hell. We know very well that the drug is an intro to other illegal drugs. For all of us, it's quite true that marijuana smoke is much more deadly than tobacco smoke to the lungs and general health, particularly when used immoderately.

Amphetamines and cocaine are similar in action on the central nervous system. They cause an explosive expenditure of those brain chemicals that we need to keep us out of depression and feeling good. Alcohol does this too, but not to the same degree or as rapidly. This is the "high" that's temporarily produced by these drugs and is so addictive. Tolerance is a problem that continues with chronic use of all drugs, requiring more and more to produce the same effect. Depression gets deeper and can even lead to suicide. Cardiac arrhythmias can occur, and some of these are fatal. I've personally resuscitated some of these in the emergency room.

Opiates tend to produce more drowsiness and a dreamlike state as well as impair judgment and willpower. You may recall that, historically, some of the European powers subverted all of China by the introduction of opium back in the Colonial age. Again, the chronic use of these drugs produces tolerance. They're effective at relieving pain and can be a wonderful aid in a chronic or terminal illness. Drug manufacturers have struggled for years to find a non-habit-forming, synthetic, opiate. So far I haven't seen much success in this endeavor. Physicians have become conditioned to the addictive properties of the opiates. They're reluctant to prescribe them, even in patients who are terminal. Obviously, this is ridiculous and I'm happy to say that this trend in pain relief seems to be reversing.

LSD doesn't seem to be with us very much anymore. That's a good thing, since it produced a temporary psychosis that tended to become more established. There are other drugs on the market, however, that produce a schizoid affect such as psilocybin and mushrooms and the amnesiacs, such as ecstasy. Even animal tranquilizers are abused, sometimes with fatal effects.

I really doubt that we old farts have much to do with the above drugs. I'm sure there are a few old pot smokers among us, having experimented with it in the 1960s. Let's face it; abusing drugs isn't compatible with living long enough to enter the hallowed halls of the elderly farthood. That would be particularly true of intravenous drug users, since they're at high risk for AIDS and hepatitis anyway.

Of much more concern to us is the abuse of prescription medications. True, some of this happens because of "doctor shopping." This occurs when one seeks care from multiple physicians unwittingly or deliberately, not bothering to tell the latest one about medications being taken as a result of a prescription from a previous one. Electronic prescribing will go a long way toward correcting this. It's been my experience that most of this happens in female patients, but that may be because women are more accustomed to seeking medical care than men. I do think that most conscientious doctors are very concerned about multiple medications and side effects. Unfortunately, there are those doctors who are known to be easy at writing prescriptions. Drug abusers tend to cluster around these, like bees around honey. These doctors usually get caught. Those who seek drugs for personal use or for resale will go to incredible efforts to try to make a valid case of injury or illness. I've seen people abrade the skin with sandpaper or deliberately burn themselves, sometimes in exotic ways, to obtain prescriptions for narcotics.

I suppose that some degree of substance abuse and drug abuse will always be with us. As a society we need to do our best to educate and rehabilitate these folks. Again, please remember that the majority of our prison inmates are incarcerated because of crimes committed while under the influence or in an effort to obtain money for the purchase of these substances. This too, is an incredible cost to society and usually is not ascribed to health care.

Chapter XVI:

Death and Dying

"Methuselah lived 900 years. Methuselah lived in 900 years, but who calls that livin' when no gal would give in to no man what's 900 years." I love that song from the opera *Porgy and Bess*. The Gershwin brothers with DuBose Heyward had an incredible ability to get right to the heart of the matter.

This isn't a fun subject. I do feel a bit of panic when thoughts of death bubble up in my consciousness. There are so many things to do, so many books to read, and so many places to go, before I depart this fair Earth. My ninety-six-year-old grandfather nailed it, though, when he said, "I don't mind dying so much, but I do hate to leave all of you."

And it's true. The most precious thing in our lives is the love and affection that we have for each other and for our family and friends. I grieve for those whose circumstances have denied them this wonder. The course of human relationships is at least as bumpy as that of true love, but, at the basic level, most of us can say that the bond that ties us together is still strong and meaningful. If we do have differences that keep us apart, I hope that we'll have the time and the desire to settle them before it's too late. Unresolved conflict takes a real toll on all of us, especially those left behind at death.

We really don't know what awaits us on the other side, do we? Is death really a transition? Is there an afterlife? The ancient Egyptians believed that there was. Over the ages, many of the philosophers and most acute thinkers felt that there was life after death. Most of the world's religions believe in this or reincarnation, in some form, as well. Is it our innate egoism that leads us to believe that something as unique as the human soul has an existence beyond the body, perhaps even coming back and recycling into another body or creature? Buddhists and Hindus believe this. An afterlife is basic to Christian theology. Near-death experiences that have been reported seem to point in the direction of an afterlife that is pleasant beyond com- prehension. But as Shakespeare puts it, "that bourne from which no traveler returns," remains a mystery.

While we expect death, as we age, we delight in others whose life span is long and hope that we will be so favored. Heredity is still the major determinant. In our present soci- ety, there are many modes of living and exposure to toxic substances such as tobacco and pollution from various sources that seriously affect us. We grieve over all death, but we're especially affected by the death of our young. Accidents remain the biggest cause of death up to the thir- ties as well as a leading cause of death in later years. Who would've believed at the onset of the automotive age that this economic engine of our society would demand the sacrifice of 50,000 or so individuals a year in our coun- try alone, plus unimaginable financial reparations?

Recently, friends lost two grandchildren in an auto accident. Their mother and another grandchild survived. The death of a child or spouse is an incredible stress. These blows seemed intolerable. How does one survive such a thing? We have no choice. We must. Not only for our family and friends, but also for our continued existence. A strong system of belief, or faith, is a big help. The support of those friends and of our remaining family helps. Things will never be the same, but we adapt, we survive. Needless to say, we learn how to survive these strong shocks from our family and close associates in our developing years. I've said it before and in different ways that isolating children from stressors such as death and funerals leaves them unprepared for tragic loss when they reach adulthood. And, we all will have it unless we die first. One of my very dear friends who has a cancer with a probable grim outcome told me recently, that he hoped to show family and friends how to face his probable demise with dignity and in a good spirit. What a guy!

For those of us trapped in debilitating, sometimes painful, illness and for those of us who are prisoners of our own bodies, death can be a welcome friend. Many times, at the bedside, I have seen the faint but clear smile of relief as a person slips away. It seems to me that medical efforts to relieve terminal pain and distress are sometimes seized upon as a potential source of wealth by a litigious society. I'm thinking of the heroic physician who stayed behind with her patients at the risk of her own life after Hurricane Katrina. She eased their suffering. She was later charged with murder. How sad! How very sad!

I would like to be wrong about this. There are doctors and other medical personnel in our health care system, who regard the death of an individual as a personal failure. This happens when those of us who are at the end of a productive life are unable to be resuscitated and brought back into an alert, comfortable, and meaningful state of existence. Is this another of those ego-driven useless mad charges into the mouths of cannon? Sometimes it's due to the misguided feelings of family members, who, when questioned will state, "Oh yes, do everything you can to keep Mother [Father/Grandma/Grandpa] alive." Alive?

Well, "everything you can do" includes chest massage to the point of breaking ribs and breastbone, inserting a breathing tube down the windpipe, placing the unfortunate one on a respirator, central IV lines, and drainage tubes in the bladder and tubes into the stomach. At that point, the loved one is isolated and sedated in an ICU without any possibility of dying with a shred of dignity and compassion, surrounded by family. We do a hell of a lot better for our beloved pets. I've heard people attempt to justify this by saying, "Well, I didn't want anybody to think that we weren't doing everything we could do keep the loved one alive, that we didn't care." Of course, at this point, the patient isn't really alive; they're vegetating. Sometimes, I've had to bite my tongue to keep from asking family, "What did this individual do to you that make you want to punish them like this?" And it is punishment; it's expensive punishment. An unbelievable amount of the health care dollar goes to this kind of terminal care. I've also heard the same family member say, "Now, I wouldn't want this done to me, of course."

Finally, one of the really good and caring things that we can do for our loved ones is to plan and organize our affairs to the extent that we can before we pass away, if we have the opportunity. We shouldn't be fools! We all know that we must die! What a fine thing to do for our survivors! It's not that hard to have a will made to make our wishes known. Getting advice from your personal attorney or trusted physician and making a health care power of attorney, is not "facing a death squad," as some of the more rabid political extremists call it. It's simply good sense. Also, a living will is a terribly important document for all of us. We need to state in no uncertain terms what we want done in the event of a stroke, severe accident with multiple injuries, severe head trauma, life-threatening infection, terminal cancer, or any other overwhelming illness. The question here is whether or not a recovery to a reasonable state of mind and quality of life is possible without resorting to lengthy, extraordinary means. This isn't always clear, even to the physician, but he or she can certainly give you the best available advice. Your prior wishes, outlined in a living will, take a great load off of your family.

Even plan your own funeral, if you wish. Not only is this your last chance to have it your way, but also you remove the considerable burden of your loved ones having to make these decisions. Thinking about it in a calm, deliberate manner sure as hell isn't going to make your demise happen any sooner.

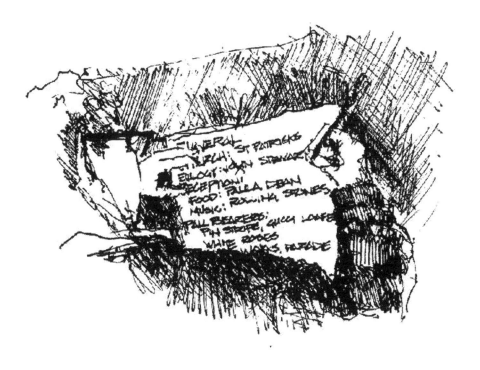

I can't leave this subject without remembering the very sweet lady whose wish was to outlive her husband so that she could take care of him at the end and make his funeral arrangements. She did this—and literally dropped dead as she was leaving the funeral home. To me, that was poetic beyond words, and a testament to true love. It was a relatively easy double funeral for the family.

Chapter XVII

Navigating the Health Care Maze

We are said to have a "system" of health care in our country. It certainly wasn't designed as such. Rather, it happened. Medicare, Medicaid, and the health care insurance industry have overlaid some semblance of system but overall, it just grew, like Topsy. It certainly is complex, especially if you're in a panic mode with an acute illness and need care. It follows, then, that a smart old fart would have a plan of care before illness comes. Men are especially bad about this. Usually, we don't have to deal with illness in our younger years and we acquire the feeling that nothing is going to happen to us that we can't handle. Again, that's called the "bull of the woods" syndrome. Don't wait till the EMT transports you to the emergency room. While the ER has protocols to follow, hopefully sorting out potential life-threatening problems, it's possible to languish there for hours.

It seems an almost futile task describing health care in this country when it's in such a state of flux. Most of the changes that are proposed have to do with means of financing health care and of determining how inclusive our system will be. Although I have my personal thoughts on these matters, I won't begin to second-guess the outcome. I suspect there will be several turbulent years ahead followed by constant revision.

The basic problems will remain at the operating level, and this is what we're going to talk about. It's of critical

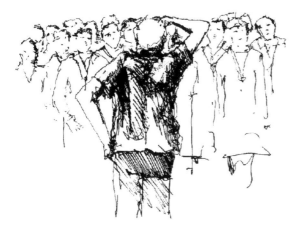

importance that you have an ongoing relationship with a personal physician, physician assistant, or nurse practitioner. Now, there are many varieties of health care providers all scrambling for a piece of the health care dollar; some of these are quite aggressive. In general, I think those individuals or groups should be avoided, particularly if they want to sell you on a course of treatment or make outlandish claims of a cure. Your practitioner should always have a relationship with an accredited hospital. You should always be informed of a provider's credentials, and these should be posted in a prominent place. You should be suspicious of degrees from an institution that can't be easily verified. The Internet is great for doing this. The American Medical Association and the various specialty societies are good sources, as well.

Medical schools graduate a lot of doctors, but numbers are not keeping up with population growth. In 2010 there were 19,392 medical and osteopathic graduates in this country. These numbers are misleading because there is (and has been for years) an imbalance between the number of doctors who can deliver primary care and the limited specialists. Well-trained primary care doctors, family physicians, general internist, ER doctors, and general pediatricians are quite capable of taking good care of 75 percent of our health problems. The ob-gyns can provide a lot of primary care for the ladies. Unfortunately, our current physician supply breaks down into about 75 percent limited specialist and 25 percent physicians capable of delivering primary care. Why are there more subspecialists? Simple: they're better paid. There are many other reasons for this imbalance, and it needs to be changed, but those are outside the purview of this discussion. You might be interested to know that just because a doctor is superbly trained in dealing with a specific area or disease, that doesn't mean that he or she is qualified in all areas of medical care, except on TV where the doc can deliver a baby then dash to the OR and do brain surgery. In fact, one of the cardinal rules of being a good physician is that of knowing your limits.

This thought is worthy of a little expansion. A primary reason for the increased cost of our medical care is the round-robin referrals that occur among limited specialists, and it happens this way: An individual selects a specialist to take care of a problem that is perceived to be within the area of the specialist's expertise. Many times this isn't the case. The specialist feels duty bound (and in some cases, financially involved) and orders several expensive tests, ultimately deciding that the problem doesn't involve his or her specialty. Then the patient is sent to a specialist in a different field, who may or may not be more appropriate, and again a series of testing takes place, which may or may not be helpful. Sometimes it's unreal how long these round-robins go on.

There is, and has been, a growing reliance on medical testing. It seems that as testing has become more effective, more of us trained as doctors are losing our abilities in physical diagnosis and examination. Add that to the seeming reluctance of medical schools to admit people who have the ability to communicate, to talk with patients, and we end up with technicians. I can't call these individuals "physicians." The most common complaint I hear about doctors is that, "He/she won't talk to me." Hey, he or she may not examine you either, but they are hell-bent on testing. You'd think that the letting of blood went out of fashion sometime in the 1800s, but not so.

Again, the primary care practitioner will know the appropriate diagnostics to perform in taking care of you. If the illness or condition is outside the practitioner's capabilities, at the very least you'll have the benefit of an informed referral to a specialist known by your doctor to do good work. One other thought here: If you can't communicate with or don't have good rapport with your primary care provider, find another one. This, too, is very basic.

The relationship between physician and patient should be private, and communication should be easy. To me, a physician is a doctor who will talk and communicate with his or her patient. I want him or her to be caring, empathetic, and give me the face time that I feel I need. I want to be able to have confidence in him or her. A doctor who has these qualities is a healer, a true physician. If you have one, count yourself lucky and value that individual accordingly. Technical expertise can be obtained, but interpersonal skills are, sadly, too rare.

We're facing a critical shortage of primary care physicians both now and in the future. There's also a chronic shortage of nursing staff as well. The nursing shortage is due to a low pay scale and the increasing use of registered personnel in administrative positions. The number of physician assistants and nurse practitioners is increasing, and this is a good thing.

To continue with your personal health care planning, you should keep a list of current medications on your person and on your refrigerator door (this per EMT protocol). "What medications are you taking?" This is among the first questions asked in the ER or in the office of another physician to whom you may be referred.

Speaking of medications, it's worthwhile saying that the prescriptions that sit on the shelf and are not taken as directed do you no good and may even cause harm. Usually, your care provider will question you about your compliance in taking your medication properly, but it can be confusing and, as I say, even dangerous when increased dosage or another medication is prescribed. Changing doctors happens, but don't bounce from one to another, particularly "forgetting" to mention your previous care! If memory is a problem, there are techniques and mechanical devices that can help you take medication as prescribed.

We citizens of the United States spend a larger portion of our resources on health care than any other nation. We should be at the very highest levels of health and good medical care in the world. This is true in some key areas, but generally speaking, several other countries are ahead of us in health and longevity. Now, we do have some personal responsibility for this. Obesity, tobacco use, and low levels of physical activity are mostly personal choice, at least outside of childhood.

Health care insurance, like other insurance, evolved as a way to spread risk. Health care has become an impossible burden for us as a society. As we well know, it can and does bankrupt individuals. Insurance programs such as Blue Cross and Blue Shield evolved to help protect us from these tremendous costs. Unfortunately, in providing reimbursement for medical and surgical care and hospital costs, insurance has become a major contributor to the rampant health care inflation that's now crippling our society.

Initially Blue Cross and Blue Shield and possibly some others were mutual companies in that their policyholders owned them. They were and still are regulated by state insurance commissioners. Sensing a lucrative opportunity, private companies entered the health care field. Some mutual companies, even some of the Blues, have become private, for-profit entities. Rapacious entrepreneurs then make fortunes, and the public subscribers pay the price. Profit in and of itself is one of the foundations of our society. Granted, those who work in the health care field are entitled to a reasonable wage, but is it right and proper to make excessive profits for investors out of illness? Or for insurance and health care executives to make obscene salaries? Or for some surgeons and technical specialists to receive extravagant fees on the back of human misery? I am a physician who is an old fart. When I began practice almost fifty years ago, my charge for an office call was four dollars. Believe me; I could rant on about this for hours.

Remarkably, instead of spreading the risk, the health care insurers seek to avoid risk. They won't ensure chronic illness or those who are at high risk for expensive care. They deny and delay payment of claims. They control enormous financial resources. They're quick to feed off of unwary government programs, and have developed tremendous influence in Congress. If the value of investments drops, the insured are quickly pressed to make up the shortfall with higher premiums. Hopefully, recent changes in regulations and the delivery of health care will stop some of this gouging.

Here I go again. Obviously, I feel that it's unconscionable to profit from illness. Certainly, physicians and those who deliver health care are entitled to fair income. They invest years in education and training. Their responsibility is incredible.

Hospitals must stay open. But, here, again, many hospitals have become private investment tools and must yield that big profit. Even nonprofit community hospitals put large amounts of money into a profit. Here it's called "operating reserves" or "endowment." Administration has exploded. An emeritus professor at a prominent medical school recently looked out over a large clinic associated with the school and remarked that 20 percent of the staff was giving care and 80 percent of the staff was "suits." Well, that's the horse we're riding at present. All I can say is, where possible, vote for change.

How do we get affordable health insurance to tide us over until we're eligible for Medicare? The really fortunate will have retirement plans that include health care. Here are some suggestions:

- Plan on getting as high a deductible as you can manage.
- Set up a health care savings account. This may be tax deductible.
- Ask your health care providers and hospitals which companies have the least denials for payment.
- Be aware that some insurance companies will drop you if you have a large claim or serious illness. This appears to be changing by law, but check with your friends and look for websites.
- Avoid highly advertised plans or those with unsolicited mailings.

What follows is very important! A health care will and power of attorney can save a lot of grief for you and your family. It should contain your wishes about how much and what is to be done if you have an accident, a cardiac event, a stroke, or other illness requiring unusual care or resuscitation and you're unable to make decisions about your care. Think of resuscitation as a fancy word for what is to be done when and under what circumstances. Do you want the EMTs and the ER to do CPR? Do you want to be on a respirator, and, if so, when should it be stopped? Do you want a feeding tube placed down your esophagus, or directly into your stomach? Do you want to prolong IV fluids? It's a terrible burden to have family members agonizing over this kind of care in a moment of crisis. Again, all too frequently, loved ones will say, "Oh, do everything you can."

I know I don't want to end my life dwindling away in a vegetative state for weeks or months. I'm reasonably sure that you wouldn't want it either. I don't really think the family wants it, but, again, perhaps afraid of being thought of as not caring enough, they will utter these words. At this point, the health care team is obliged to go through the motions, even though they know that survival isn't likely or that the quality of life possibly gained simply isn't worth it. You are now aware that a very large percentage of the health care dollar goes toward end-of-life care in this manner. Last word in this chapter: Execute that health care will and power of attorney. Again, hospitals can help you with this, so can your attorney. It absolutely should be done before it's needed. Keep a copy available for the squad; for your health record at the doctor's office; and on file in the hospital record, if you have one. Certainly, make it known to your significant other, who should also participate in drawing these documents up, if possible. Again, make sure that you have a regular will and even plan your funeral.

Personally, I hereby direct my survivors to have a party instead of a wake or a "viewing" at the funeral home. I want them to have fun, to celebrate my overcoming mistakes and rejoice in any triumphs. We did this at my beloved maternal grandmother's funeral. All of us remember that get-together and the fun we had with her. I'm sure that "Miss Bessie" was smiling right along with us.

Chapter XVIII:

Be Careful, Others Are Watching...

Well, where is this chapter going? Don't worry; it's not in the vein of *1984*. I recently had the opportunity to read my fifteen-year-old grandson's school essay concerning his visit with us last summer, during which we built a small boat (he got an A).

His memoir was a lot more detailed than was my memory. Oh, it was me, all right! Now I recall, tossing a new hammer into the creek in anger when I couldn't drive a nail straight with it. New hammers are like that sometimes. The old one, with a wooden handle, worked much better.

The point, though, is that my grandson was soaking it all in. My feelings, my mood, my language, my impatience—everything. Children do this to perfection. They constantly seek clues as to how they should react when faced with similar situations. This process starts when they're born, maybe before. Obviously a parent has much more influence just because of exposure time, but never discount the intensity with which a grandchild observes you.

Of course, everything goes into the mix. Teachers, store clerks, doctors, nurses, police, firefighters. Yes! It does take a village; it takes a village of people who are kind, giving, considerate, slow to anger, helpful to others, loving, kind to animals, honest, hardworking, and unselfish—all the good qualities we'd like to have ourselves. And, of course, we'd

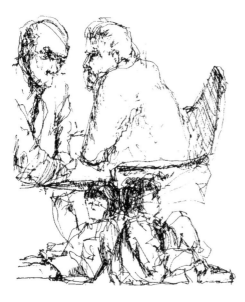

like to pass this on to our progeny. But, all too often, we go negative, and find it hard to see good in anything.

I have a friend like that. Once he gets down on something, he never misses an opportunity to slam it. Isn't much fun to be around him anymore. He hasn't always been a downer, and I wonder what happened. I do think that many of us, as we get older, have a tendency to get cranky. After all, when we look around, there are plenty of things to be cranky about. There are unfortunate wars, the economy, the political situation, taxes, rising medical costs, and even the rising costs of funerals, not to mention gasoline. I could be a curmudgeon at very short notice. Fortunately, my dear wife yanks me back to sanity before I get too far down this line. She's right, of course. There's no benefit to be had from being down on everything. We actually make ourselves depressed and become less able to cope—and less fun to be with.

I remember a backseat conversation among two eight- or nine-year-old boys while we were driving to a beach vacation. One of these guys was my son. The subject was family visits and how they hated them. One boy, freckle faced and redhead,said that after they kiss you on the mouth (ugh!) the old women sat around in a circle and talked about their operations and how bad everything was now, particularly in the younger generation, and how they just didn't know how they were going to get along. And each woman tried to make her situation worse than the others'. You can imagine this banter between youngsters at that age. We in the front seat had to bite our lips to keep from laughing, and to hear what was coming next. We really don't have license to let it all hang out as we reach these exalted years.

Our grandkids are watching us. Grandma's cranky, but she's just getting old, and that reminds me of another story from years ago when I made house calls. It was an elderly couple that sat in adjoining rooms. Obviously, this had been going on for years. It was like a tennis match. Instead of rackets and balls back and forth, they hurled frequent barbed comments and insults to each other. They were in their eighties. After I got over the shock, it was almost entertaining. Their children were in anxious attendance. I don't remember what the medical problems were at the time. They did die, not long after, and oddly enough, within two weeks of each other. They obviously were close in some rather weird emotional sense. The next two generations of the family that I knew of were dysfunctional, but perhaps no worse than some.

Chapter XIX:

Family, Friends, and Faith

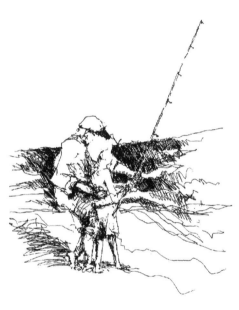

We can't get away from them, even if we wanted to, and most of us don't. Quite the opposite, we will change locations to be closer to children, and especially grandchildren. At the same time, we can get somewhat selfish with our time and privacy. Then, of course, we end up feeling guilty. One of the first things infants learn, spontaneously, is the art of making a parent feel guilty. How in the world does this happen? But then, even our pets manage to learn this.

I'm not thinking of more desperate situations where a grandparent is left as sole support of a grandchild or has to babysit regularly for a single parent when the child's parent must work. These things we do without even a second thought. Frequently, though, when grandparents are close by, their babysitting talents can be overused, even demanded. That doesn't happen without one's permission, of course.

We love our children, but we love and adore our grandchildren, and that can lead to problems. I remember one family where the grandparents were rather wealthy and owned an auto dealership. Among many other things, they gave a grandson a new car. This kid, for kicks, put the car in reverse and did backward circles until the transmission was shot—whereupon his doting grandparents immediately gave him another new vehicle without a murmur. Now what kind of lesson did the kid get from that?

We might think that we can buy their love and affection, but we lose their respect when we become pushovers. Then, we can no longer advise and counsel, making use of the experience and wisdom that we hope has evolved with these advancing years.

A problem that frequently surfaces too late to do much about is that of a child or grandchild who doesn't come to visit or spend time with you. How frustrating! Now, finally, when you have the time to give, they aren't around to receive it. But, wait a minute! Could the problem be in the phrase "now, finally, when you have time to give"? Remember, children learn by example. When they were small and needy, did you give them time? Or were you just "too busy"? There's a great country song with this theme. It may not be too late for you to correct your relationship with the grandchildren. You're fortunate beyond words if you have a close relationship with your children. (By the way, this includes nieces and nephews and their progeny as well.) I think one of the more severe problems faced by our society is the breakdown of the extended family.

Another common problem in our relationships with family and friends occurs when we have disagreements or arguments that we are unable to bring to a resolution. This can be due to almost anything. Frequently they are trivial. Many times these misunderstandings have their deeper origins in old incidents that are forgotten. The sad thing about these hostilities is that they are very destructive. They don't hurt the people against whom they are directed, necessarily, but they do turn inward on the person holding the grudge. Sometimes these grudges are mutual, sometimes not. But they're destructive, nonetheless.

I will continue to state that the most wonderful thing in life, the thing that's most valuable any way you want to measure it, is the love and affection that is possible among and between families and friends. I think that as we get older and recognize our mortality we begin to sense this. What a shame, then, to allow these hostilities to continue. They deprive us of the joy that might be ours. And it's a real tragedy when the other individual, parent, sibling, or friend dies, leaving the problem unresolved. Then it becomes like a cancer. It's worth almost anything one can think of to forgive and forget, and to communicate this to the other party. I've seen people hold on to a hurt or a grudge until their entire life becomes defined by it.

A friend is a most wonderful thing to have. One of the older truisms is that if in the course of your lifetime you make one good friend, have the trust and affection of children and of a good dog, you've done pretty well in life. Some of us are fortunate enough to have our spouse as a best friend and confidant. This is truly the hallmark of a close and trusting relationship. As long as we keep communication open and try to avoid the pettiness that can eat away at everyday happiness, we're well on our way toward maintaining these relationships. Some of us are better than others in making and keeping friends. While all my siblings are good about this, one brother is especially so. I've noticed that he makes an extra effort to remember little things, to help his friends out, and maintain communication. I wish that I had been more diligent in looking after my friends. So many times I have put that letter aside, or waited too long to answer a phone call, or for that matter, to make one. I still regret that I did not look in on my old medical school dean and his wife, a much revered couple, who had retired near to my home. Too late now!

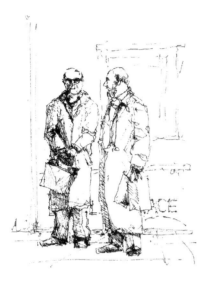

What I'm saying here is that having and maintaining good social relationships with friends and family is an essential ingredient in the quality of our lives, certainly in health and longevity. Anger, hostility, and isolation are not compatible with a long and happy life. You choose!

Many of us are fortunate enough to have really elderly parents, aunts, and uncles alive and reasonably well. Unfortunately, many of our highly mobile families are split up by geography as well as by divorce. Caring for a parent or other elderly relative can be difficult and sometimes impossible. There are many factors at play here. Not only health, but also resources, dementia, and sometimes just downright stubbornness come into play. These are tough problems to deal with. We become fiercely protective of our independence, particularly driving a vehicle, as we advance in age. My paternal grandfather at ninety-four was most upset when the family hired a seventy-five-year-old cousin to stay with him as a companion. "That boy don't know nothin'!" was his retort. The relationship didn't last and Grandpa spent his last two years in a nursing home. Sometimes, all one can do is work the situation with loving firmness; but don't be surprised if that doesn't work either. Of course, there are assisted-living facilities with all levels of care, including those with full nursing care. They may not be for everyone, but, hey, whatever works.

After all, there may come a time when we need help and care personally. This is where planning comes in. A health care power of attorney is essential. A personal power of attorney is good for a trusted family member to have in case of sudden and unforeseen disabilities, temporary or permanent. And no matter what assets you have or possessions you've accumulated, if you have a will it can avoid a lot of scrambling and ill will among your survivors. I think most of us like to have the last word. This is the way you do it! I know that I've said this before and I'll say it again. It's that important! Go online or get legal help as a resource.

It's great if we can and will work out our own elder care plan and have it in place when needed. Naturally, those of us who have the care, concern, and resources to do this for our family are the ones least likely to need it. We hate to consider disability, much less death, but planning for it sure as hell doesn't bring it on any sooner.

Faith

And now, allow me just a brief step into the subject of faith. Most of us have some level of faith in our makeup. Personally, I don't feel that it matters much as to what system this faith is involved with. We're more comfortable, more at ease, and healthier when we have faith in something. Of course, there are many: Judaism, Christianity, Buddhism, and Islam, even atheism. They're all good, and in very large part have the same tenets. The problem comes when extremists pick out those parts of doctrine that support their wild beliefs and undertake to act on them by punishing those who don't agree with their fanatic interpretations. Most of us in this world no longer believe in stoning or punishment by mutilation or torture, for example.

What really works is our joining together with like-minded people in a system of worship. If we do believe that we have a soul, this is good for it. Tolerance and caring for those less fortunate or ill are all positive features and, again, are found in most systems of faith. Where would we be without those organizations that exist for the purpose of disaster relief and help for our unfortunates in this manner? Afterlife? Who knows? I would rather believe the positive than the negative, given the circumstances. Meanwhile, enjoy the satisfaction of making the world we have into the best place we can!

Chapter XX

Retirement

When we're young, retirement seems far off. We think we're never going to live that long and are not quite sure that we want to. Well, guess what? It's here. We made it, for better or worse! Of course, that depends on current economic conditions as well as our personal lives.

Retirement itself really is a mixed bag. To begin with, many of us are having so much fun working that we don't want to quit. I know quite a few physicians, for example, whose lives are so ingrained in their work that they don't want to consider a life without it. There's nothing wrong with this. There are multiple reasons at play here, any one of which is adequate to support continuing that lifestyle. Sometimes it is helpful to shift the focus of one's work while remaining in the same field. This brings new incentives and pleasure to the task.

Another thought; sometimes it's more appropriate, and satisfying to quit while at the top of one's game. It is sort of sad to let ourselves wither on the vine, losing our abilities and competence. Of course, it's very hard to be objective about this. Many of us are very reluctant to give up positions of power and prominence, if we are fortunate enough to have them. It must be easier for the professional athlete whose declining abilities are very apparent to coaching staff, as well as the public. And as you know, some organizations build in age limitations on continuing to work. Unfortunately, this is usually a process of "one-size-fits-all".

Our current economic environment brings many of us to another decision. We are financially unable to retire, or at least to retire in the manner to which we had hoped to become accustomed. So very many things have occurred to bring this about. There is the decrease in property values, residential as well as commercial. The cost of educating our children at universities and in advanced degrees has risen exorbitantly. When these things are coupled with global recession, it can become quite necessary to continue a job when we have one or to seek additional employment. Many of us, who are already retired, have been forced to go into lower paying work in order to supplement our retirement. In general, though, I think our generation is willing to do whatever we have to do in order to survive a rough spot. Another way to look at it, we're better off with something to do than sitting around watching television and bemoaning our fate. It certainly is healthier.

Those of us who are retired are frequently questioned by those who want to retire or have plans to do so. At least they're asking about it. Questions can cover any aspect of retirement, but the most frequent is, "What do you find to do?" Right away you know that this person is in for a tough time. Assuming one has a choice, under the circumstances it might be better to continue to work. All of us hear the stories about people who quit work, retire, or just stop doing anything, and fall over a few months later with a heart attack or stroke. This seems to happen more with males who are wrapped up with their jobs and have little, if any, outside interests or hobbies. Until recent times this hasn't been as much of a problem for women because they've been and continue to be employed as homemakers, frequently in addition to public jobs. Also, they have more diverse interests that they can call on throughout life.

At times one hears, "I've worked hard all my life so far, and when I retire I'm not going to strike another lick!" If this is you, you're in real trouble. Just like any other mecha-

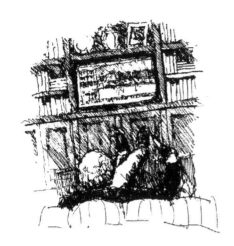

nism, we'll rust out before we wear out. One of my cousins was employed as an executive in a major corporation with good benefits some years ago. He said that when he retired he was going to sit on the sofa, his wife on one arm and a bottle of beer in hand and just "fat myself to death!" A young man's boast, but as an old man he achieved his goal. His last years were not healthy ones. Fortunately, he had dementia.

It's really difficult to avoid our Puritan work ethic, or at least keep it under control. We tend to value ourselves by the yardsticks of achievement and accomplishment. We don't seem to realize that there are lots of other yardsticks out there. There's an almost endless list of volunteer work available to us that can contribute incredible value to society and in turn to our lives. Think of it—volunteers are valued everywhere! Hospitals, nursing homes, schools, organizations that do volunteer consultation for small businesses, and even as EMTs. And, of course, there's Eldercorps and other organizations, religious and charitable, that give aid and disaster relief in this and other countries.

We must plan for life after our children are grown and, hopefully, gone. Hobbies are wonderful and can be absorbing as well as fulfilling. Educational opportunities for elders abound and are frequently coupled with travel. Many retirees become experts in their field of interest and consult and write articles in various specialties. Teaching is great and can be a second career if one wants. My college roommate taught economics at the university level for nearly 20 years after retiring as a Navy captain. Our public school systems need all the help we can give them. I can't think of a more worthwhile endeavor than giving back to the society from which you came or contributing to society in underdeveloped regions of the world.

My wife says that I do much better—and am even easier to live with—when I have a schedule, official or not. A few years ago, I really enjoyed taking a wooden boat-building course at a local community college. I got my butt out of bed at six in the morning and attended five days a week for a year and a half. I really felt great! I lost weight (not as much snacking), improved my woodworking skills to a high degree, built a beautiful boat, and still have a nice sense of accomplishment from that. I wonder if I have time to build that thirty-foot schooner after I finish my "honey do" list?

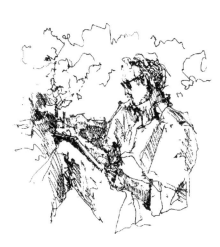

Like a lot of us, I tend to procrastinate or get plain lazy if I don't have a schedule. But, make it yourself; we resent having a schedule imposed on us, and probably wouldn't keep it anyway.

You may think it's too late to find a hobby or something to do if you haven't done it before retirement, but, if you want to speed up the aging process, do nothing, nada, zilch!

Chapter XXI:

Transportation and Travel

It's been said that we the people in the United States rank our freedom to drive an automobile very high on our scale of privilege. Truly, we do love our ability to hop in a vehicle and go anywhere from the corner drugstore to cross-country. Our society is built around the automobile, to a large extent. Many of us can continue this activity well into our advancing years, but there are cautions. We, as individuals, and those around us need to stay aware of those limitations that creep up on us. We don't want to become a danger to ourselves or others. Sure, I know of some individuals driving—even flying a private plane—into their eighties and nineties. We're very jealous of these prerogatives and tend to overestimate our abilities in order to preserve them.

What are some of the danger signs? We're all aware that the ability to respond quickly to a changing situation fades as we age. Turning, braking, avoiding a person, avoiding a creature or object, the simple act of turning your head to look out of the side or rear mirrors—all of this becomes more difficult. Episodes of confusion or loss of awareness are certainly major concerns. I've said to my children and grandchildren over the years that "situational awareness" is one of the best protective modes we can be in when driving, operating machinery, or even walking. In my woodworking shop, I try to be constantly aware of where my fingers are when operating a machine. So far, I still have ten.

I remember one situation where the husband had lost a lot of his mental capacity as he aged. He'd been the family driver for years. His wife retained her smarts, but had never learned to drive. However, she was the instructor par excellence. "Turn left here! Now turn right! Stop!" They managed, but not too well. After several accidents—fortunately, none fatal or causing serious injury—and after driving through the garage wall, they gave up their keys. Even though we resent someone telling us that we're no longer safe to drive, we need more frequent testing to make sure we remain safe. Private pilots are tested every two years, no matter what the age. I simply can't imagine the sorrow of living with the knowledge that I'd caused serious injury or death because of driving with impairment from any cause.

Many times, one hears the story that family members are hesitant to restrict or stop the driving privileges of older family members. They should not be bashful about this, nor should you feel resentful if it happens. If they don't do it, and know that they should have, they become complicit in any accident that occurs. Remember, it doesn't matter whether the accident is your fault or not. A good driver can avoid many accidents because of a quick reaction time. Still, its hell to have to give up this very important aspect of our independence, but the possible alternative can be a lot worse.

Before leaving the automobile, it's worthwhile to talk about a few problems that we can develop and ways to avoid them. Getting sleepy is certainly one of the most dangerous. Even drifting off for a couple of seconds can be tragic. Pull off to the side of the road. Get out of the vehicle walk around. Make use of the rest stops. Again,one should stop and get out of the vehicle every two hours to prevent blood clots forming in the legs. This does happen. Most of us remember a prominent correspondent who died in this manner after riding in a cramped position in a military vehicle for some time. He wasn't all that old, either.

There are other alternatives. Metropolitan transit always has provisions for its older customers. Sometimes these are even on call. And many times, friends or family members are available to accompany us or take us to the doctor, dentist, or grocery store. Then, there's always a taxi. This isn't demeaning; it's just good sense.

One doesn't have to be restricted to his or her home area, either. There are many cruises, bus tours, and guided vacations available. Many of these are specifically aimed at us older folks. Although some of these require a reasonable ability to move around and walk, some can accommodate wheelchairs or walkers. But a frequent objection I've heard from my contemporaries is, "I don't want to be pinned up with a bunch of old folks on a tour!" And that's worth thinking about for a minute. Do you constantly talk about your illnesses, operations, and bowels? Do you whine about your arthritis, family, and loneliness? (This tendency has jovially been called an "organ recital.") If this is you, you may not be much fun to be around in a social setting. Try to be more concerned about current affairs and the interests of our companions. Listen more! Talk less! Do not whine! Remember Abraham Lincoln, "I had rather be thought an idiot than to open my mouth and remove all doubt."

I don't know about you, but as I age I find myself getting more anxious about air and train travel. Am I at the right gate? Do I have plenty of time? Should I have carried my luggage? Incidentally, I always carry a kit containing my medications and toiletries with me. I've even been known to carry extra underwear.

All of the airlines, tours, and most modes of travel are eagerly seeking your business. They're quite willing to provide assistance when needed. One merely has to ask.

By far the best thing, though, is to have a knowledgeable traveling companion. Of course, experience is great.

The more you travel, the better off you are. The more accomplished you become, the less anxiety you have. The introversion, that all of us experience to a varying degree as the years go by, makes us even less likely to travel. Sometimes, I will try to turn down a trip because of anxiety and concern or just the plain trouble of getting it together and going. I've always had fun and enjoyed the trip, even when I'm pushed to go. After all, a desire to travel is almost universal with us. We do like to see different places and things and experience different cultures. All through life, we tell ourselves that when we retire or when we have time, we want to travel. Do it while you still can, and especially when you can do so with your significant other.

Chapter XXII:

Pets

Now, I can almost hear some of you saying, "Hey, wait a minute. Is this guy really writing about something as insignificant as house pets?" Well, guess what, buddy? It's been proven that we who have pets live longer and are healthier than those of you who don't want to bother. So, there!

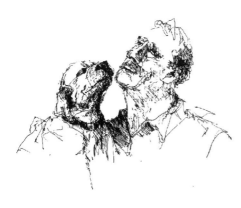

As a pet owner, I certainly admit to a great deal of prejudice toward the comfort and companionship of having a pet in your house. I'm going to discuss dogs and cats, not only since they are the most common pets, but because they're able to return affection usually to a greater degree than that which they are given. Sure, turtles, snakes, iguanas, birds, and fish have their place. They do indeed represent an entity to which care and affection is given, and that is important also.

The relationship between humans and dogs and cats has existed for many, many thousands of years. It's been commented on all throughout the literary genre and studied a great deal in scientific literature. You can't help but wonder just how the relationship came about. Was it the availability of food? Perhaps it was a warm fire, shelter, and the affectionate scratching of a tummy. Maybe it was praise with a kind voice. It was probably all of the above. The ability to hunt and to rid a dwelling of vermin was certainly a plus from the human standpoint. We were even willing to put up with fleas, but we probably had them in plentiful supply anyway, along with lice.

It is well known that loneliness is debilitating for almost all of us. There's no question that we are healthier and live longer when we have a pet. Sure, we'll complain about the time and effort and expense of looking after a critter, but the mere action of having to look after something or somebody is important to us.

Let me diverge a bit here and remember many instances wherein an individual was devoting a large amount of time and psychic energy, as well as work, to caring for a sick or elderly partner or relative, or, for that matter, an invalid family member. When the equation changed and that level of care was no longer necessary, usually because of death, then the caregiver would go into some manner of withdrawal. I've always thought of it as having an unexpected surplus of psychic energy. It has to be used up somehow, whether diverted into other caregiving or volunteering, or it'll cause problems.

I have had people tell me that they've had pets and enjoyed them, but then the pet died and the loss was terrible. They just didn't want to go through that again. We all have a tendency to avoid being hurt if we can. But I tell these folks that if you do not allow yourself to be vulnerable to being hurt or sad, then you automatically cut off any chance to experience the joy and comfort that a pet can give you. The same thing applies to human relationships, of course. My wife and I went through serious grief when we had to put down our Great Dane, Capt. Jack, because of illness at nine years of age. We still miss him deeply, talk about him a lot, and look at his photos. But, we simply couldn't do without the tremendous love and affection that we gave and received from that super guy. A few weeks later, we rescued Molly, another Dane, who is at my feet as I write this. It's a lot like having another individual in the house. It's very comforting, to me especially, as my wife travels a lot for her work. Sure, I have to provide food and water, scoop poop (make that big poop), take her for walks, and learn her version of dog language (she has certainly learned a lot of mine). I know that this is good for me. Mark Twain had several good quotes about dogs, one of which was, "I don't want to go to any heaven that doesn't have dogs." Somebody else said that dogs were the only creatures that you can feed and be kind to that won't turn around and bite you. I defy you to look into the eyes of a dog and not see kindness and love, even if the dog isn't your own.

It's remarkable that these pets are so finely attuned to our feelings and moods. Not only are they very sensitive to our personal situation, but also they're very much aware of the ambience of the household in which they live. Again, using Molly as an example, we rescued her from a divorce situation, which was somewhat intense, as you might imagine. We were told that she had skin problems, and, indeed, her hair was sparse in certain areas and there was a good deal of dandruff-like flaking of the skin; a veterinarian was treating this. After taking her to our home we neglected to do anything about it for a few days, and, lo and behold, the condition completely resolved. Neurodermatitis?... In a dog?... You bet! Another thing: When my wife and I are in an "intense" discussion and I'm getting the worst of it (I nearly always do), Molly will come and sit or lie down by my feet. I'm sure that all of us know of similar incidents; I think I could relate them for hours.

Oh, I have to tell you about this one. The morning of 9/11, I was sleeping late, but got up to let Capt. Jack out for his morning pee. Shortly, I heard a soft howl. This was unusual for Jack. No fire or police sirens were tuned up, no other dogs were vocalizing, and I wasn't playing the harmonica or singing. Puzzled, I got up and turned on the television to the view of the disastrous first Trade Center collision and, to my everlasting horror, saw the second, and then saw the buildings collapse. Now, we live several hundred miles away from New York City, and while I didn't witness any similar howling during later events, I'm reluctant to dismiss this as an accident. You know the old saying from Hamlet, "There are things in heaven and earth, Horatio, undreamt of in your philosophies." I'll leave it there.

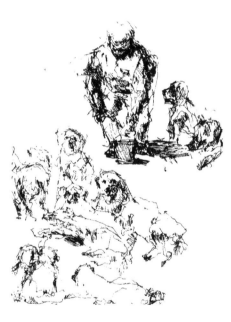

Another thing: I have nourished the presumption that one wanted to get a dog or cat as a puppy or kitten. The thinking was that the puppy or kitten would develop a closer bond to its owner. The tough side of that, which is really not all that bad, is house or litter box training and going through the gnawing and destructive stage that the young ones go through. After rescuing Molly as a fourteen-month-old, we have no reservations as to the degree of love and affection an older animal gives us. Do consider adoption if you'd like a pet. These critters are so happy to be adopted and cared for. I don't think anything is sadder than an abandoned dog or cat. (By the way, it's my personal feeling that cats should be indoor critters. Outside, they are highly destructive to songbirds and other small life and they turn feral easily. Now, if one has a barn full of rats and mice, that's another matter.)

The dog, and to some extent the cat, don't love us " because." If we give them any kind of basic care and a little affection, they just love us, and we love them. And, this is a healthy thing. Again, it has been proven that people who have pets live longer. I know that they're happier too.

Chapter XXIII:

Living Solo

Some of us want to live alone, get away by ourselves. Many of us endure circumstances that force us to live alone. I suspect a lot of us that do live alone would rather not. It's certainly a situation that happens. It may not be too good for the fainthearted.

But suppose you're one of those who never married. Perhaps you've been a widower for a while. Under these circumstances, one is forced to develop routines and skills to carry on. Families can be a big help here. Of course, they can only do so much. After all, they have their own occupations, their own lives to live and their own families to care for. Frequently they are living in an area too far distant to be of any consistent help. They'll be worried, of course.

In these situations, it is very nice to have good neighbors and to stay in contact with them. Again, I will talk about my mother-in-law, who is living alone in her nineties. She has several good neighbors in the condominiums where she lives. Even though these ladies are considerably younger, they have fun cooking for each other and going shopping occasionally, or out to a movie. This wouldn't work if she were cranky and reclusive. I would say that if you're not a companionable person you're going to be in trouble.

Most communities have a lot of opportunity for social occasions. Most educational institutions welcome the attendance of older people. Some have special classes

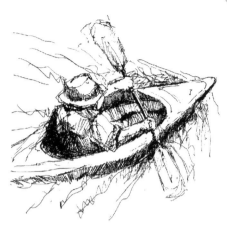

for you. There are numerous clubs, some having to do with hobbies, some civic. Most churches make a point of looking in on their older members, especially if they are known to be living alone. We must remember that we are a social species. Most of us do better when we have the companionship of a group.

At the same time, there are many things to be said for solo living. You make your own decisions, good or bad. Of course, you can just drift along with the current and accept whatever comes your way. You do your own chores. You cook, you clean, you wash the dishes, and you do the grocery shopping. Or you can just let everything go to hell. You can watch television all day and all night, if you wish. Or you can read all day and all night, if you wish. Or as the old song goes, "I eat when I'm hungry, and I drink when I'm dry."

Unless you're experienced with solitude, you're very likely to have trouble adapting to it. I know many older men who've been so babied and cared for that they're unable to prepare anything to eat, much less clean up or wash the dishes. They can't even pack for a trip. This is really a helpless situation and guaranteed to put the individual into a tailspin when a separation or death occurs.

I was talking, recently, to a friend whose wife had died not so long ago. "How are you making out? "Well, not too bad! lonesome as hell, of course". " I can imagine. Good to see you still singing in our community chorus ." "Oh, I stay busy keeping up with household chores, bills, and all that stuff. I'm even getting to be a pretty good cook." "You

WILLIAM B. WADDELL, MD

mean you didn't do any of that before? " "No, but I was fortunate in that we had a couple of years together after the diagnosis and my wife put me through a training course." What a warm loving relationship that must have been!

Many of us are not the best at organization, much less establishing a routine and sticking to it.

I was the oldest kid in our family. I had two younger brothers and, a good bit later, a sister. Somewhere about age ten, my mother, picking up on a bit of interest I had in the kitchen at the time (I liked food even then), told me that she was going to teach me to look after myself. In retrospect, I recall that she said nothing about looking after my siblings, but at age 10 I wasn't terribly analytical. As I recall, she said something like, "I don't want you to have to depend on some durned old girl to look after you." So I was taught to cook, clean up, and wash dishes, and could even run a washing machine. Now, my mom had always worked in the office with my physician father, and in essence had become his office nurse. In those early days, we did have a nanny, but as we got older we became latchkey kids. We all had our share of chores, which included attending to the victory garden and looking after the chicken lot. In the Depression years, house calls, home deliveries, and sometimes office visits were swapped out with produce and livestock. In any event, this all worked out for the good in that all of us grew up as fairly self-sufficient individuals.

Personally, I love food and enjoy cooking. Fairly often, I'll have dinner prepared when my wife gets home from work, is tired, and wants to sit and relax for a bit. She also enjoys cooking and is developing a reputation as a gourmet cook. At these times, she runs me out of the kitchen. My contribution comes afterward in cleaning up and doing the dishes.

Well, I've digressed a bit here. Improving one's cooking skills really isn't too difficult. There are an incredible numbers of cookbooks and food magazines available encompassing all skill levels. Following a recipe is easy enough. Once you learn what ingredients go together, you can begin to freewheel quite a lot. When my wife is out of town, I would rather cook for myself than go out to eat. It's not that I don't like good restaurant meals; I do, but not as a steady diet. Forget fast food. There's not much that's healthy or all that tasty there. The cheap stuff is starch and other carbohydrates, fats, and sugar, and a lot of them. Sure, I've been known to scout out a really great hot dog or hamburger or a great plate of eastern North Carolina barbecue, but, hey, after I pass age ninety-five, all bets are off. I'll try to keep my weight down, but I'm sure not going to worry about cholesterol. Arteries that aren't clogged up by then are going to have to make out the best they can!

Perhaps the most insidious thing that happens when we live alone is the involution, or folding in, of our person-alities. We begin to lose interest in current events and our friends and family. After a while, our circle of awareness and interest decreases, getting smaller and smaller, and we end up as a candidate for assisted living or a nursing home. A lot of dementia seems to originate in this fash-ion. I can't say it enough, we're social individuals, and we function better in a social setting. We need the stimulation of conversation, of good books, music, art, and, most of all, friendship.

There's another insidious and dangerous side effect of solo living. This is increased alcohol consumption. How very easy it is to watch some of the mindless television that we have, for example, and reach for another glass of scotch or bourbon or make another martini, sometimes forget-ting how much we've already had. Older people do not tolerate the effects of alcohol as well as they did when younger. It doesn't take as much to seriously affect coor-dination and balance. Falling becomes more likely. We fall asleep in the recliner, or in the bed and the days and nights hurry by. Combine this with the smoker's curse, and you're lighting the fuse of a fire that can take you beyond all caring.

Since we tend to be social critters, one might think that some manner of communal living would work out as we get older. This becomes far from easy. It is perhaps best when we can have separate dwellings, but still have proximity to fellow elders. Not only do we have our own developed habits, likes, and dislikes, but also we find it difficult to accommodate those of others in a close situation. I think women adapt to this much easier than men do.

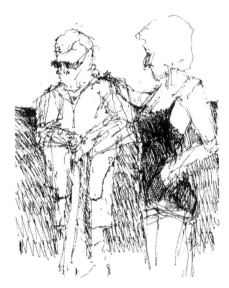 I will say one more time that we need companionship... Many of us will dive into another relationship after a loss. The warmth of sitting with your significant other reading or watching TV can be very comforting. Being able to share your thoughts and ideas and to have a conversation, the level of which rises above grunts and wheezes, is wonderful. Traveling without a companion isn't a lot of fun for most of us. If you're able to achieve this closeness in a living situation, be very thankful and value it accordingly.

There seems to be a larger number of older men on the lookout for women who are caregivers than there are women searching for someone to care for. There's nothing wrong with the caregiving scenario as long as people are honest with each other and each willing to contribute to the relationship. I don't think I need to say that sexual activity among elders will be a primary consideration. Of course, one should realize that there are many levels and varieties of sexual activity. This is nice when it happens, though.